Connected Lives

Families, Households, Health and Care in South Africa

Edited by Nolwazi Mkhwanazi & Lenore Manderson

Published by HSRC Press
Private Bag X9182, Cape Town 8000, South Africa
www.hsrcpress.ac.za

First published 2020

ISBN (soft cover) 978-0-7969-2585-5
ISBN (pdf) 978-0-7969-2586-2

Copy-edited by Patricia Myers-Smith
Typeset by Nazley Samsodien
Cover design by Conor Ralphs
Photo credit (inside back cover): Masimba Sasa
Printed by Capitil Press, Paarden Eiland, South Africa

Distributed in Africa by Blue Weaver
Tel: +27 (0) 21 701 4477 | Fax Local: +27 (0) 21 701 7302 | Fax International: 0927865242139
www.blueweaver.co.za

Distributed in Europe and the United Kingdom by Eurospan Distribution Services (EDS)
Tel: +44 (0) 17 6760 4972 | Fax: +44 (0) 17 6760 1640
www.eurospanbookstore.com

Distributed in United States, Canada and Asia except China, Lynne Rienner Publishers, Inc.
Tel: +1 303 444-6684 | Fax: +001 303 444-0824 | Email: cservice@rienner.com
www.rienner.com

Suggested citation: Mkhwanazi N and Manderson L (eds) (2020) *Connected Lives: Families, Households,
Health and Care in South Africa*. Cape Town: HSRC Press

Contents

Preface

The family as a powerful network of relations of care, and the household as a setting for the production of health, together influence everyday life, health, wellbeing and care in contemporary South Africa. Yet little attention is paid to the historical and contemporary diversity in family, household size and household composition in many policy statements, much public discourse, and many research publications on families and households. The following all point to diversity and flux in relation to partnership, parenting and residency: local traditions of polygamy and instances of powerful men with multiple wives; contemporary rhetoric relating to low rates of marriage and to single-headed households; and the Constitution of the Republic of South Africa (hereafter 'the Constitution'), which protects the rights of people regardless of sexuality. Yet people still speak and write as if the small nuclear family is normative in South Africa to the same degree as it is in the Global North. Diversity is typically framed as a sign of dysfunction, but, as we illustrate in this book, families and households function, nurture, thrive and provide resilience under all kinds of circumstances.

In an article published in the journal *Medical Anthropology*, Nolwazi Mkhwanazi (2016) drew on Chimamanda Ngozi Adichie's critique of a 'single' story, and called on researchers to take this as a serious challenge in scholarly work. Lenore Manderson and Susan Levine (2018) extended this, arguing that theory from the Global South could not be realised without supporting, acknowledging, drawing on and finding inspiration in research from the South. Further, we need to nurture our own researchers, and to do this, we need also to teach from the South. This book aims to advance this project. We have used a structure that illustrates the extensive work of South African scholars and other researchers conducting research in South Africa. Much of this work, especially that of younger scholars, is in the form of master's and doctoral dissertations, and few people outside these scholars' home institutions have had an opportunity to engage with it. Other work has been written up in the 'grey' literature – reports from government and NGOs (non-governmental organisations) – which is rarely cited in international publications (largely in the Global North). We feel strongly that the outputs of this work need to be read and taught. The case studies in this book largely derive from this work, and offer unique portraits; around each case study, we weave a narrative of how families care, to illustrate the diversity and disrupt notions of a singular way of life.

This book had its genesis at a workshop on Kinship and Families of Care, which Lenore Manderson convened with Ellen Block and Hylton White in March 2015.

At this meeting, several researchers working in South Africa and neighbouring countries on families and care presented their ethnographic and population-based research on reproduction, care and dependence, and we began to explore the subtle and more explicit ways in which families generate, assemble and re-form at key points in the life course and in response to serious life events. In this context, we observed, conventional idioms of kinship and family at times obscured relationships, responsibilities, affect and personal economies.

This meeting resulted in two special issues of journals. For the journal *AIDS Care: Psychological and Socio-medical Aspects of AIDS/HIV* Lenore Manderson, Ellen Block and Nolwazi Mkhwanazi (2016) edited a supplement entitled *Responsibility, Intimacy and Care*, which highlights the challenges to giving and receiving care, particularly among poor and marginalised populations, and the limits of health-system and legal responses to these challenges. And for *Social Dynamics* a special issue, *Kinship and Constellations of Care*, was edited by Lenore Manderson and Ellen Block (2016a; see also Manderson & Block 2016b). It provides a comparative account of changes to families, including the increase of single-parent, female-headed households and nuclear families, and the creative ways that enable people to take on everyday and higher needs for caregiving.

Our interest in furthering interdisciplinary collaboration in this area, and in bringing together interests related to family and household, health and care, led to another workshop at the University of the Witwatersrand in September 2016, and a further two-day workshop in March 2017 on Families, Households, Health and Care. Both these workshops were supported by the DST-NRF Centre of Excellence in Human Development based at the University of the Witwatersrand. Many authors contributing to this book participated in these or earlier meetings (senior and emerging researchers, from government research agencies – particularly the Human Sciences Research Council (HSRC) – and various universities and departments). Other case-study authors were invited to contribute to the book, and in some cases we worked with them. The authors come from a wide range of scholarly disciplines, including psychology, sociology, anthropology, public health, community health and demography. This is reflected in the methods that informed their case studies – surveys, ethnographic research, interviews and intervention research. The case studies are all based on larger studies by these researchers, and we have provided references to allow readers to explore further the context, methods and ethics of particular studies.

In the case studies, the names of all people are pseudonyms, so as to protect the privacy of individuals. Place names are real unless otherwise indicated. As was noted above, the case studies included in this book provide the empirical evidence to illustrate the concepts and general observations that we discuss in the integrating text; they were selected to reflect some of the diversity of family, households, health and care in South Africa. However, we capture only *some* of the diversity.

Race, sexual and gender identity, and class all impact on family life and household composition, but very few case studies are concerned with white, coloured or Asian families; only one article is concerned explicitly with gay South Africans, and none is concerned with queer families (for this, see Morison, Lynch & Reddy 2019). This points to the gaps in scholarship and the need for more research, and we hope that our narrative and those of the case-study authors point to the directions in which such research might go.

We do not conceive of the book's structure as static: we see multiple ways in which it can be read and used as a text. The case studies have been incorporated into chapters to illustrate specific themes, but – as will become evident – there are other ways of organising the material and thinking about content. Further, as we discuss in Chapter 1, the majority of case studies, although emanating from various provinces, regions and home settings, concern African women and men. The absences draw attention to the need for further work on households and families.

Numerous grants bodies and universities made our own work and our collaborations possible. In particular, Nolwazi Mkhwanazi thanks the DST-NRF Centre of Excellence in Human Development for funding the research for her case study, and the National Institute for Social Sciences for funding the research for the case study by Lebohang Masango. She also acknowledges the University of Global Health Equity, Rwanda, which provided the space that enabled the completion of the book. Lenore Manderson is grateful to the DST-NRF Centre of Excellence in Human Development for its support for the workshops held in 2016 and 2017, from which developed the structure and content of the book. She thanks the Centre too for its support of some of the research that informed her writing.

We thank the HSRC Press for responding with grace and enthusiasm to our proposal, for its commitment to seeing the book to press in a timely manner, and for the excellent copy-editing indexing and design. We thank also the Humanities Faculty Research Committee, the School of Public Health and the DST-NRF Centre of Excellence for supporting the publication of the book.

Over the years the two of us have worked at the intersections of medical anthropology, public health and gender studies. We have built a network of academic support and we are thankful to our colleagues for their support of this endeavour. Nolwazi Mkhwanazi is especially grateful to Naledi Mokoena and Deevia Bhana for their collegiality; Lenore Manderson to her colleagues and students, across continents, whose work most closely shaped her appreciation of the themes that we address. We are indebted to the contributing authors for embracing the challenge with which they were presented – to write short, compelling accounts that would allow readers into the lives of the people with whom they worked. We thrived, too, on the challenge to pursue our ideas on diversity. And in realising this shared project, we also thank each other.

Nolwazi Mkhwanazi and Lenore Manderson

Johannesburg, 15 November 2019

Abbreviations and acronyms

AMA	Advanced maternal age
ART	Antiretroviral therapy
ARVs	Antiretrovirals
C-section	Caesarean section
CSG	Child Support Grant
DoE	Department of Education
DoH	Department of Health
F	Female
HBR	Hated But Respected (gang)
HSRC	Human Sciences Research Council
KZN	KwaZulu-Natal Province
LGBTIQA	Lesbian, gay, bisexual, transgender, intersex, queer, or asexual
LMICs	Low- and middle-income countries
LSA	Learner Support Agent
M	Male
MMR	Maternal mortality ratio
MOU	Midwife-run obstetric unit
NGO	Non-governmental organisation
NIDA	National Institute on Drug Abuse
OP	Organophosphate poisoning
RXH	Red Cross War Memorial Children's Hospital
SABMR	South African Bone Marrow Registry
Stats SA	Statistics South Africa
STI	Sexually transmitted infection
UNAIDS	Joint United Nations Programme on AIDS/HIV
UNIFEM	United Nations Development Fund for Women
WHO	World Health Organization

1 Changing family structures and everyday relationships of care

Lenore Manderson and Nolwazi Mkhwanazi

At a meeting held in Johannesburg in March 2017, Tawanda Makusha spoke of the complexity and variety of households in a peri-urban area of Pietermaritzburg. Household sizes varied from 1 or 2 to 29 inhabitants – some households had contracted over time, others were extremely large and stable, others swelled and shrank according to circumstance and time of year. Happenstance can shape household size, and who does what within it, every bit as much as cultural norms around tradition, love, marriage and responsibility for infants and small children.

The *South African Child Gauge 2018* (Hall et al. 2018) includes six types of household in South Arica. The most common type is the extended family (36 per cent); then the single-person household, with only one household member (22 per cent); then the childed couple, incorporating a couple (married or not married) and a child or children (19 per cent). The lone parent residing with their own children and no other adults makes up 11 per cent; couples residing alone make up 10 per cent of households; and the composite family – any household with at least one unrelated member – makes up 2 per cent of households. While surveys can be problematic because of how the information is derived, this information from the *South African Child Gauge 2018* does provide some indication of dominant living arrangements and the extent to which they deviate from the supposed norm of the nuclear family. Further, household composition and size do not necessarily indicate stability, and over time households expand or contract with births, marriages, fostering and adoption, migration and deaths. Usually, but not always, households include family members, and some include people who share a space for practical reasons; other households become de facto families, even if the relationships through blood and marriage – consanguinal and affinal ties – are tenuous. Regardless, households provide both the context of everyday living, and the labour involved in sustaining health and wellbeing. At the same time, families extend beyond households, locally and at greater distance, with variations in the strength of the ties of family members and their involvement in each other's lives. These are major motifs in the chapters, and the case studies, that follow.

Various factors have influenced household composition and impacted on kinship relations in South Africa. Among these have been punitive political systems; laws and institutions; population politics that countered human rights; economic precarity; personal conflict; and high levels of migration for work (Button et al. 2018). Writing about the second generation of isiXhosa-speaking communities of the Eastern Cape townships in the 1960s, BA Pauw (1963) explained the high numbers of matrifocal families as the result of a combination of migrancy and high rates of illegitimacy. He highlighted the difficulty for an unmarried mother and her children living in a township to be completely independent as a family, especially with regard to childcare. However, if an unmarried mother lived with her mother, thus attaining 'the three generational stage', then independence was possible (Pauw 1963: 148).

Families, however constituted, are the most important social support structures for all people worldwide, regardless of a country's economic status; degree of industrialisation; and the structure, size and provisions of the service sector. Affective social ties bring meaning to people's lives. The power of family relationships is not replaced in any setting, even when some of the work of a family is, or might be, outsourced by, for example, childcare or aged care, domestic workers or live-in assistants, takeaway food and meals-on-wheels, or community health workers and volunteers. Such services and support systems are provided on both voluntary and commercial bases. They are designed to meet the needs of families and households where appropriate support can no longer be provided within the household, and where individual and household wealth, community organisation, or healthcare systems can meet these needs. The ongoing transformations of living arrangements impact on household capacity to meet the need for the everyday care of household members, as well as added needs that derive from responses to health crises, acute illnesses, chronic disease, and challenges associated with multimorbidity and caregiving.

In South Africa, the structure of households was shaped indelibly by nineteenth- and twentieth-century practices of colonisation, labour migration and apartheid. But in the twenty-first century further factors disrupted families and gender relations. Among these were structural changes; economic shifts; and seasonal, temporary and long-term migration (Bocquier et al. 2014; Collinson et al. 2014; Madhavan & Schatz 2007); and decimation from AIDS (Comaroff 1985; Schatz et al. 2011; Schatz et al. 2012; Schatz et al. 2015; Schatz & Seeley 2015). At the same time, gender norms continue to dictate women's and men's roles, at least normatively. Women are seen as the caretakers of the homestead, bearing and rearing children, undertaking domestic productive activities, and caring for the ill and frail. Men are seen as responsible for generating income. Economic and social forces continue to drive working-age adults to migrate. Many people find employment as unskilled labourers or find contract and seasonal employment on commercial farms (citrus farms, sugar plantations, and so on) or in agricultural packhouses, but there is a continued and growing flow of people moving from rural areas to cities, especially Johannesburg, in search of paid employment (Posel & Marx 2013; Smit 2001). Increasingly, these immigrants are women. Many of these internal migrants, and men and women particularly from neighbouring countries, live on the streets, and are socially isolated and vulnerable (Schenck & Blaauw 2018).

As the *South African Child Gauge 2018* illustrates, a substantial number of female-headed households exist for various reasons, and the number has increased over time (Hall & Mokomane 2018: 38). These households experience greater poverty and hardship than households of married couples (Rogan 2013), partly due to gender disparities in income. Nevertheless, women in South Africa are much less likely to remarry than women elsewhere in southern Africa. This partly reflects high levels of gender discord: intimate partner violence is extremely high in South Africa, with nearly 30 per cent of men said to have committed an act of rape and nearly 50 per cent physically violent to a partner (Chopra et al. 2009). Women who have suffered gender-based violence are reluctant to report and seek care outside the household, for fear of further violence and abandonment (Dunkle et al. 2004; Dunkle et al. 2006; Gari et al. 2013; Morrell et al. 2012; UNIFEM 2011). Unequal access to household resources, usually skewed towards men when there are adult men in a household, aggravates women's economic vulnerability (Hausmann-Muela et al. 2003; Merten 2008; Tanner & Vlassoff 1998; Tolhurst et al. 2008). Changes in partners, and the dissolution of marriages, also contribute to women's and children's vulnerability and household precarity.

Household structure and formal kinship ties, informal flows of resources, and entitlements and access to state grants all impact how householders manage different care needs (Schatz 2009; Schatz et al. 2012; Schatz & Ogunmefun 2007; Schatz & Seeley 2015). These factors also impact how different family members, resident or not, help to meet these needs. Government grants, as we explain, intervene for many people with low income. However, people living with limited capability or in poor health, poverty, and economic insecurity depend most on their personal networks for physical and practical support. Households of grandchildren and grandparents, or grandmothers especially, are common, either because the child's parents have migrated for work or because of death. Some households may include three or four generations of people variously related – aunts, children from different fathers, and so on. In the 1990s and early 2000s, HIV and AIDS decimated families, eroding personal networks and contributing to household poverty. Skip-generation households became increasingly common as a result, and, in consequence, older adults were expected to provide extensive care for people of various ages, even while their own health may have been compromised or declining (Gómez-Olivé et al. 2014; Schatz et al. 2015; Schatz & Madhavan 2011; Schatz & Ogunmefun 2007). Children orphaned by AIDS may be taken into care for pragmatic and pecuniary reasons (Dahl 2016) or kinship obligations (Mkhwanazi & Block 2016; Reynolds 2016); in both rural and urban environments, their care and schooling may be compromised (Raymond & Zolnikov 2018). In addition, women often leave their children in the care of others (their own mother or the child's father especially), when they migrate for work or to study (for further discussion, see mothers and grandmothers in Nairobi in Clark et al. 2018).

Gender roles everywhere influence decision-making about and patterns of caregiving and support. While gender norms in South Africa provide scripts about who is expected to provide care, largely placing responsibility on women, growing numbers of men in long-term unemployment have taken on caregiving. However, relatively little is known about what this care involves and how it is experienced (see Block & McGrath 2019). In South Africa in 2017, only 35 per cent of children lived with both their parents, 41 per cent lived with their mother and not their father, and 3 per cent lived with their father and not their mother; 20 per cent – 1 in 5 children – lived with neither parent. This means that 76 per cent (some three-quarters) of children lived with their mothers, but only 38 per cent (just over one-third) lived with their fathers (Hall & Mokomane 2018: 37–38). One reason for fathers not living with their children is breakdowns in relationships; other reasons include poverty, migration and unemployment. Even so, fathers may keep in contact with their children and contribute financially and personally in their upbringing. Further, if the father is completely absent, children may have other male authority figures who live with them, or whom they see regularly, and whom they may regard as fathers (Van den Berg & Makusha 2018).

In this book, we are concerned with how households and families are constituted, and we explore how, in different households, people care for each other, for infants and small children, and for the sick and elderly. We examine how people manage tasks and challenges within families and households on an everyday basis, while they negotiate constraints, competing needs and demands. We consider how people care for themselves and others with complex health problems under conditions of changing personal and economic circumstances; varied employment opportunities; and shifts in gender roles, flows of resources, and decision-making and authority. The state plays an important role in supporting households and families, too, under a variety of circumstances, as we describe further below. Although the cash value of the grants from the state is relatively small, households are at times constituted around them (Patel et al. 2017a; Roelen at al. 2017).

Regulating health and realising care

Public health policies, innovations in medical technology, effective medications and improved access to them, and improvements in living conditions have in most countries in Africa, and globally, led to reduced mortality, higher life expectancy, and increased ageing. In South Africa, as elsewhere, people are living longer, with now-treatable conditions and increased access to and affordability of effective treatments. With the scaling-up of antiretroviral treatment, for example, South Africa now has one of the highest numbers of people living with HIV in the world (Shisana et al. 2014; Stats SA 2016), and people are able to live full lives as a result. Concurrently the prevalence of cardiometabolic diseases – obesity, diabetes and cardiovascular disease – is high, accounting for 20 per cent of mortality (Clark, Gómez-Olivé et al. 2015; Levitt et al. 2011). These health conditions – like all changes in health and illness – are managed firstly within households, supported by the free provision by the government of essential medicines, including for HIV, TB, cardiovascular disease and diabetes. At the same time, there is growing emphasis on self-care and home management of illness, with limited external support. The South African government, like governments of other states, expects that families will provide a secure environment for themselves and their children, and manage HIV and other chronic diseases. These trends converge and are intertwined. Household members and family members must balance care needs and demands against immediate economic needs and opportunities, time and cash constraints, and long-term considerations, including in relation to the education and long-term wellbeing and security of children (Dahl 2016; Golomski 2016).

Communities and families, in rural settings especially, interact with existing formal social-protection schemes, providing the personal support structures for the care of children and household resilience (Shenderovich et al. 2018; Steinert et al. 2018), for the prevention and treatment of chronic conditions and the health and wellbeing of community members on a continuing basis. While community health workers often provide critical support and supplement others' efforts (Nxumalo et al. 2016), the life-long management of HIV and other chronic conditions is household based. The everyday care of people living with disabling conditions, including mental health conditions, and people who are aged and frail (Deist & Greeff 2017; Kohler et al. 2018; also see Braathen & Swartz's case study 6.3 in Chapter 6 of this book) also impacts on others in households and among a wider kin network. Such care extends from meeting direct costs – including those associated with transport, with medical advice, and with obtaining, filling and adhering to prescribed medication – to supporting dietary and other changes, to within-household decision-making associated with changes in health status and challenges in disease management. Such care also includes variations in need for assistance, according to a person's ability to maintain everyday personal care (cooking, bathing, toileting), and whether a householder has multiple health conditions, medication and care regimes. How everyday life unfolds varies between households. For example, the everyday life of a household experiencing economic pressures, but with no members who have chronic health conditions, unfolds differently from that of a household centred, at least to some extent, on a person with high or demanding care needs. In the latter case, various householders and non-resident kin – and to some extent non-kin neighbours – are involved in decision-making, assistance, contributions of time and finances, and support (as Viljoen, Myburg and Reynolds's case study 5.5 in Chapter 5 of this book illustrates).

Unemployment, single parenthood, disability and older age all influence individuals' capacity to meet their own needs economically and physically, and the South African grants system provides financial support to individuals according to various criteria. A number of different grants are available to support individuals and, through them, households and families. The Child Support Grant (CSG), most frequently mentioned in this book, is payable to the parent or primary caregiver of a child or children living with the caregiver and under the age of 18. The Care Dependency Grant provides support for children born with special care needs; it is paid until they reach the age of 18. The Disability Grant is paid to people from 18 to 59 years of age who, because of a mental or physical disability, are unable to work. At 60 years, recipients of this grant, and all older people, are eligible for the Older Person's Grant (or old-age pension). People who fought in a world war or the Korean War are entitled to apply for a War Veteran's Grant, although few people now qualify and the grant is essentially fungible with the Older Person's Grant. People who need full-time personal care, and are receiving either the Disability Grant or the Older Person's Grant, are also eligible for a Grant in Aid to pay the person responsible for providing full-time care; this grant is not means tested. Finally, a Foster Child Grant is paid to foster parents while the child is living with them; this grant is also not subject to a means test. The case studies in this book highlight the pervasiveness of state support in people's everyday lives and caregiving contexts. The sizes of the grants are relatively small. In August 2019, as we finalised this book, the amounts were R410 per month for a Grant in Aid; R420 for the Child Support Grant; R1 000 for the Foster Child Grant; R1 780 for the Care Dependency, Disability and Older Person's grants, and R1 790 for the War Veteran's Grant. In addition, a further grant, the Social Relief Grant, can be made for a period of three months in specific contexts, including when other grants are being processed. The grants are often the only regular income stream for a household and provide motivation for people to live together.

In these contexts, kinship rules, obligations and understandings vary on the basis of social and economic exigencies, the resilience of households in relation to such conditions, and the capacity of people to manage chronic health conditions in the context of structural vulnerability and entrenched poverty. The poor health of individuals of productive age may especially influence household and family wellbeing. (In rural areas with high unemployment rates, many households rely on grants; in this context, loss of the income-generating capacity of people of productive age may not have great impact.) These challenges are most likely felt at an individual level, or by households of relatively small size, in urban settings and in informal settlements, where people may not know and may be wary of neighbours, or may have few friends or other family members to whom they might turn, and where communities are fragmented, if they exist at all (Madhavan et al. 2018; Raniga and Mthembu 2017). Such challenges are especially marked for people who have migrated from other countries (see Musariri and Moyer's case study 6.4 in Chapter 6).

In this book, we explore contemporary changes in family-making and household structure, and economic and care arrangements, and we show how household composition and kinship relations influence decisions regarding caregiving and support. In the case studies included in each chapter, we consider the shifts and exigencies that impact on decisions and have practical consequences as households change and families converge and dissipate. As we illustrate, the high proportion of single-parent, female-headed households means that relatively few healthy householders take on everyday, higher-need care of co-resident young children – including grandchildren and other minors – frail older people, and others. Further, intra- and extra-familial care relationships and resources within households and among households connected through family ties affect the health status of people with poor health and complex care needs. They also impact more generally on how health and wellbeing are produced and maintained in households, on where children are raised, on where people are nursed, if severely ill, where those with chronic illnesses are monitored, and on where people may go to seek help and care from kin (Clark et al. 2018).

Among Africans, cultural practices and values continue to play a strong role in shaping intimate relationships and family life, and because a number of the case studies refer to these, we shall discuss them here. The first is *inhlawulo,* usually glossed as compensation. This is the payment of damages from a man's family to a woman's, when that woman conceives outside a recognised union. The successful negotiation of *inhlawulo* allows for the acknowledgement of the child as belonging to the father's lineage, so clarifying – in the patrilineal systems of the region – who their ancestors are. This has important implications for the cultural identity of children, as illustrated by Mkhwanazi's case study 2.1 in Chapter 2, in Pillay's case study 3.2 in Chapter 3 and in Chapter 4, including in Mvune and Bhana's case study 4.1 in that chapter. This does not imply that the father's kin should care for the child, but it does create for the father and his kin opportunities to visit the child; such opportunities may be withheld in the absence of acknowledgement of the child's lineage. The negotiation of *inhlawulo* also allows for discussion about how to compensate the woman's family or contribute to the costs of caring for their daughter and her child. Given high rates of unemployment and persistent poverty, the negotiation of *inhlawulo* remains common, even if payment is usually sporadic. However, increasingly, over the past decade or so, the families of daughters who are pregnant have not negotiated the payment of *inhlawulo,* but instead have emphasised the acknowledgement of paternity to secure and legitimise the child's place in the patrilineage (see also Nduna & Jewkes 2012).

The payment of *lobola* or bride wealth, particularly among Zulu South Africans, is also an important convention (Posel et al. 2011; Rudwick & Posel 2015; Shope 2006). The payment of *lobola* formalises a union and confers respect on women. Unemployment has extended the time it might take for a man to generate the money to negotiate and formalise marriage ties. In consequence, as instanced in a number of the case studies in this book, men and women cohabit and have children together well before *lobola* is finalised. Historically, the payment of *lobola* arguably gave men authority over women, but it also gave to women's families the right to intervene in family affairs and so protected women, to a degree, from abuse and neglect. At the same time, *lobola* redistributed scarce resources, establishing relations of reciprocity across lineages.

Ubuntu is a central concept in African moral philosophy, throughout southern Africa and beyond. Ubuntu privileges interdependence of humans and the nature of social relationships. Roughly glossed as 'I am because we are' or 'a person is a person through others', ubuntu describes collective solidarity and communalism, mutual respect and responsibility, humility, solidarity and caring. These values ideally define the nature of relationships at local levels – that is, within communities – and at the level of the state (Kamwangamalu 1999; Metz 2011). In a number of case studies, including 5.2 (by Hochfeld, Chiba and Patel, in Chapter 5) and 6.3 (by Braathen and Swartz, in Chapter 6), the authors refer to ubuntu to highlight the sense of responsibility and mutuality that people have regarding each other; the concept also underpins the motivations of people in caring for each other discussed throughout Chapter 7.

In this book, we illustrate the flexibility of kinship, households and families in contemporary South Africa, and draw attention to the emerging differences between idealised notions of kinship and family and everyday practices of care.

Most of the case studies in this book focus on African families and households. This was not our explicit intention, but Africans comprise 80 per cent of the population of South Africa. Furthermore, the legacy of apartheid – under which legislation was introduced to fragment families and disrupt family life – is still evident today, and much of the published research on families is concerned with populations most affected by apartheid. Despite the idealistic attempts of the government to reduce inequality within the healthcare system, there are still marked differences by race in the incidence of diseases, and Africans experience worse health outcomes and poorer access to healthcare than other populations (Coovadia et al. 2009). Apartheid's legacy continues to shape African people's experiences of reproduction and reproductive healthcare; dominant ideas about gender roles; how families come to be; and how households are created. These issues are at the heart of how individuals, families and households in South Africa are connected or disconnected.

2 *Making families*

Nolwazi Mkhwanazi and Lenore Manderson

Having a child is an important event for most women. Seldom an event that happens in a vacuum, the birth of a child creates networks of relatedness through lineage and through people – kin and others – who choose to be part of the child's life. Most women aspire to have children and see this as an important mark of adult womanhood. In this chapter, we explore women's aspirations to have children, ideas about timely reproduction, and women's experiences of pregnancy and birth.

Fertility is one measure of a country's health. The term 'fertility rate' refers to the number of children born to a woman over her lifetime. High fertility rates can be problematic because a high number of pregnancies and births can negatively impact a woman's health, placing pressure on government services and infrastructure for health, education, housing and employment. Poor families, especially, may lack sufficient resources to provide their children with physical care and to clothe, feed and educate them. The South African state provides grants, for example the Child Support Grant (CSG), to poor families, and this often the only income that these families have (see case studies 3.2, 4.3, 5.2, 5.4, 6.3 and 6.5). However, as was described in Chapter 1, the monthly amount is usually too low to enable a family to make ends meet. Very low fertility rates also create difficulties, including in relation to caregiving, and nation states with low fertility rates often provide incentives to women to have more children. In South Africa, according to mid-year estimates by Statistics South Africa (Stats SA), in 2019 the total fertility rate was 2.32 children per woman, a decline from 2.62 in 2009 (Stats SA 2019: 1).

Childbirth is not always a happy occasion. The birth of some children is more valued than the birth of others, depending on sex and race of the child, and the socioeconomic circumstances, class, sexual orientation and nationality of the mother (Colen 1986; Ginsburg & Rapp 1995). The preference for some births (and children) over others has a long history in South Africa. Population policies during apartheid encouraged white women, regardless of class or nationality, to have many children in order to increase the population of the white minority. African women were discouraged from having children and were subjected to birth control measures. Today discrimination centres on age, citizenship and sexual orientation. Teenaged girls (13–19 years old), women over the age of 37, and immigrant women are discouraged from having children. For the teenaged girls, the reasoning is that the mother and the child are at an increased risk for adverse outcomes – educational, health and so on. For migrant women, the issue is one of resources; migrants are portrayed as draining the already overstretched public healthcare system. Sexual orientation does not absolutely preclude reproduction, but women without male partners are largely excluded from assisted reproduction services; in general, Nina Botha (2016) emphasises, such services are the privilege of white, middle-class, heteronormative couples. While adoption is possible, adoption agencies likewise give clear preference to heterosexual couples (Lynch & Maree 2013).

In South Africa, most people have firm perceptions about who should have children, where, when and how many. Although a growing number of women chose not to have children, the majority do. Some children are planned, others are not; and most children are cared for within families, whether biological, adoptive or foster families. For those children not included from birth in an existing family, who are abandoned or otherwise in need of care, both the state and various NGOs (non-governmental organisations) provide institutional care. However, this should not imply that the state 'cares' for these infants and children; women, and occasionally men, are hired by the state to do care work.

The first case study (2.1) focuses on a African teenaged girl, her experience of pregnancy and becoming a mother, and her family's response to this. Nolwazi Mkhwanazi draws on ethnographic data collected in 2016, and highlights the various arrangements that exist to care for children born to very young women, many still at school. In South Africa, high rates of teenage fertility cause much concern for government officials and NGOs (Panday et al. 2009; Macleod & Tracey 2010). The rates of teenage childbearing have steadily decreased (Mkhwanazi 2017), and with the introduction of new legislation and youth-driven programmes (such as the She Conquers campaign), rates may decline further. For now, however, teenaged mothers remain a visible part of the social fabric of life in poor African and coloured communities, and less so in Indian and white communities.

Case study 2.1

The complexity of care in young families

Nolwazi Mkhwanazi

One cold July evening in 2011, as she was preparing to get into the bath, Ntombi heard her cellphone ring. She was not used to receiving calls in the evening. The phone screen showed that it was her daughter, Thandi.

'Hello?'

'Hi Ma, how are you?' Thandi responded.

'I am fine. How is school?'

'Ma, there is something I need to tell you—' Thandi began hesitantly.

'Wait, before you tell me … your sister has been acting strange lately. At night she wakes up crying and asking where your baby is. What is that about?'

'Ma, I am pregnant,' Thandi muttered under her breath.

''Scuse me, what?'

'I don't understand why she is doing that. Ma, is she going to be okay?'

'What did you just say?'

'Ma, I am seven months pregnant.'

'Oh. Ok.' Ntombi hung up the phone.

A few minutes later, Thandi's phone rang. It was Ntombi.

'HOW COULD YOU DO THIS?' Ntombi screamed into the receiver. 'How could you do this to *me*? How could you be so stupid? I knew that I should never have let you stay at that woman's place. She is always trying to sabotage everything. Nothing good can come from her!'

'Ma, you either accept it or you don't,' Thandi managed to say through her tears. 'There is nothing I can do about it now.' She hung up.

Thandi's grandmother, Thoko – actually Thandi's grandfather's second wife – was her primary caregiver. Ntombi never got over her parents' separation, and she blamed Thoko for creating divisions within her family, as Thandi explained:

> My mom hates my step-gran to the extent that she said she mustn't even
> come to her funeral. That's deep. So my mom doesn't like my grandmother
> and my mother does not get along with her sister because her sister speaks
> to my grandmother. My aunt (mother's sister) appreciates the fact that
> my grandmother raised me. As soon as my granddad passed away, my
> grandmother could have been like, 'Everyone just take your children and
> leave my house,' but she raised me. She is still doing things for me now.
> She is raising my mom's grandchild! You'd think as a human being you
> would be grateful, no matter what she did to your mother. She raised your
> child and is raising your grandchild right now. Something my mom was
> not able to do and no one blamed her for it.

When Ntombi became pregnant in her early twenties, she hid her pregnancy for as long as she could, then told everyone that the father of the baby had been shot. When Thandi was a few months old, Ntombi moved to Johannesburg, leaving her daughter with her father and Thoko. Ntombi's father died when Thandi was two years old. Thoko continued to care for Thandi.

In Johannesburg, Ntombi had two daughters – Gloria, who is now 20 years old, and Thabi, aged 8 years – each with different fathers. When we met, Thandi, too, had been living in Johannesburg for over a year and had not seen her mother for three years. Her mother had never met her daughter, Omphile, who was at the time six years old.

When a young woman has a child outside a recognised union, decisions made about who will care for the child have consequences, not only for the composition of households but also for relationships within and between generations. Ntombi's anger when she heard that her daughter was pregnant was not unusual (see also Mjwara & Maharaj 2018; Naidoo et al. 2019). Nor was it unusual for Thoko to become the primary caregiver – of both Ntombi's daughter and Thandi's daughter. Decisions made about the care of children born to young mothers are at once both straightforward and enormously complex, expressing the fragility and strength of kinship bonds.

Thandi became pregnant a few weeks before she turned 17 years old. To usher in the new year, Thandi and her childhood friends in Kimberley met up with some boys from the neighbourhood and hung out, drinking in a nearby park. Thandi did not drink alcohol, and when Tshepo, a boy she had known for a few years, offered her a drink, she refused. He pleaded with her to taste the 'Red Square, Blue Ice' because she would like it. She acquiesced, and accepted a first bottle. While drinking the second bottle, Thandi started to feel drowsy, and began to nod off. Her friends teased her, saying that it was only 6 o'clock in the evening and the night was still young.

Thandi woke up the next day in the home of a friend, aching. She thought that she might be experiencing a hangover. She could not remember anything that happened after the second bottle of Red Square, Blue Ice. When she asked her friends, they told her that they had left her in the living room 'making out' with Tshepo. She did not remember this. A few days after this incident, Thandi told her grandmother, a nurse, that she did not feel well.

The feeling of foreboding disappeared in mid-January when Thandi returned to boarding school in Bloemfontein, where she was reunited with her high school friends and back in the routine of schoolwork and sports. One day in March, however, her netball teacher commented that she was gaining weight and, given how active she was, this shouldn't be the case. Her friends suggested that she go to the clinic to make sure that she was not pregnant.

Thandi's response: 'I didn't believe them because my friends knew I was a virgin. So I was like, "Am I giving birth to Jesus? Is this the dawn of a new age?" '

A few weeks later, the headmistress of the school approached Thandi, told her that she had booked her off school for the day and that she was going to have a pregnancy test. On finding out that she was pregnant, Thandi made calls 'to every hospital in Bloem [Bloemfontein] to find out which hospital could do an abortion at five months since the last time I kissed a boy was five months ago. I found one and I asked the headmistress not to tell my gran yet; I would tell her myself. It was Wednesday and my appointment was on Friday.'

That evening, Thandi's grandmother called and told Thandi that she had spoken to the headmistress. They had agreed that Thandi come home immediately, and Thoko had organised for someone to collect her the next day. Thandi protested, asking to spend a few more days because she had an important appointment on Friday. Sensing what this was, her grandmother told her not to terminate the pregnancy, but to wait until they had discussed it:

> I said, 'Okay.' My grandmother said, 'You have me and you have your aunt –' 'Wait!' I said, 'Did you tell my aunt?' And there in the background I heard my aunt saying, 'Hi.' I get home [the next day] and it is a feast. My aunt and my grandmother have cooked. There are cupcakes … There is everything. At that point, as much as this [the pregnancy] would change my life, it was a beautiful moment for me to see them like that … You don't find out that you are pregnant and then your gran and your aunt are *that* excited! So I figured God wants this, if I was meant to have an abortion I would have found out earlier.

Thandi could not remember the circumstances of conception, and so she feigned tiredness to avoid talking with Thoko. That evening, when she was in her room, Thandi called Tshepo:

> I said, 'You were the last boy that I kissed. What happened?'
>
> He's like, 'You don't remember?'
>
> 'Would I be asking?'
>
> Then he told me, 'We had sex.'
>
> I said, 'Okay, why? Why didn't you use a condom?'
>
> 'I dunno.'
>
> I'm like, 'Okay, well, I am pregnant.'
>
> He says, 'Are you sure?'
>
> I am like, 'You *did* know I was a virgin.'
>
> He was like, 'Oh yeah, I could feel.'
>
> Wow, what an arsehole!

After a moment of silence Thandi continued,

> Okay, but I feel it is not rape because I was actually aware of most things that were going on. But I said to him, 'Couldn't you wait until I wasn't in that state? Unless this is something you did on purpose.' Tshepo's response was, 'Oh shit, this is my third child.'

Thandi never told her grandmother about these circumstances. She was afraid that Thoko would press charges against Tshepo. She also said she did not want her daughter to think that she was conceived from rape: 'I wouldn't wish that upon anyone.' Instead, she told her grandmother that she had had some alcohol and 'one thing led to another.' Thoko wrote a letter to Tshepo's family, stating that Thandi's family wanted nothing from Tshepo's family except that they 'acknowledge that there is a child and if there have to be ceremonies [in the future], that they will introduce her [the child] to the ancestors as their child.' After receiving the letter, Tshepo's mother called Thandi, and while on the phone, confirmed that her son had had sex with Thandi and that he had not used a condom. Tshepo's mother suggested that they wait until the child was born before deciding what to do. But although Thandi's family were clear that they wanted nothing but acknowledgement from Tshepo's family that Tshepo was the genitor, the mother visited and brought blankets and clothes for the baby. No negotiations were made for paying *inhlawulo*.

While non-payment of *inhlawulo* may ensure stability, security and continuity of maternal kinship care for the child, this may also lead to discord and conflict within the maternal family. In Thandi's case, conflict arose because Thandi was raised by her grandmother, whom she regards as her mother. Thandi trusts and feels obliged to let her 'mother-grandmother' help her care for her own daughter.

Who cares for a child is often contested. Although Ntombi was angry with Thandi when she learnt of the pregnancy, she became excited about becoming a grandmother and being able to care for the baby: 'My mom wanted it to be a boy because she has three girls. She (my mom) just said. "If it is a boy, I am taking that kid. I am raising that child." My gran needed it to be a girl, because if it was a boy, my mom threatened to take him.'

Thandi gave birth to a girl, who she called Omphile. Even so, Ntombi wanted to be the new child's guardian:

> Every single time we talk on the phone, she tells me how my daughter must come and stay this side [in Johannesburg] and she will raise her. But ... my daughter is secure now. I know she is safe where she is. My grandmother is doing a great job raising her. If I bring her this side, me and my mom hardly see each other. Me and my mom fight a lot. I don't want to put my daughter in that. She is still too young.

Thandi was apprehensive about Ntombi's claims to her daughter. She pointed out that Thoko had been very generous and deserved the family that she had created and nurtured. Thandi described Thoko as 'quite amazing', a 'superwoman', dependable and deeply caring. This was in stark contrast to how she spoke about her mother and their relationship as 'complicated' and conflictual.

Thandi emphasised Ntombi's and Thoko's responses to her pregnancy. Her mother's reaction was one of anger; her grandmother had been calm, pragmatic and supportive. In illustrating this, Thandi recalled how she and Thoko were on their way to the gynaecologist for a check up at eight months into the pregnancy. Thoko asked Thandi if she had thought of any names. Thandi told her that at school, her peers had named the child 'Blessing'. Thandi continued:

> So she asks me, 'Okay, why do you want to call her Blessing?' I say, 'Because the Lord has given me blessings, Ma.' And then she just looked at me and was like, 'What?' I told her that I honestly feel like God has given me blessings. She said, 'Okay.' When we got to the gynaecologist, the doctor says, 'Do you have a name yet?' My gran gave her name in Setswana: 'Omphile Maake.' My gran is sneaky, very sneaky.

Thandi described her last month of the pregnancy as one of 'intensive care' from Thoko. Her grandmother worked in the morning but returned around 10 a.m. to check on her, bringing her yoghurt and biltong to snack on. She would return again at noon to prepare lunch. She would leave and be back at 2 p.m. to check on her and then again at 4 p.m., with each visit bringing her something to eat.

Thandi gave birth by Caesarean section (or C-section). When she returned home three days later, her grandmother and her aunt did not leave her side. 'My gran took leave off work for six months, maternity leave … everyone was there. My aunt even! My aunt took maternity leave as well. Everyone took maternity leave!' Thandi said, laughing.

A month later, Thandi returned to school to finish her Grade 11 and then her matric. She then studied business management at her grandmother's insistence to further her education. In Thandi's third year of studies, Thoko told her that she could no longer afford to pay for both her and Omphile, and asked Thandi to find a part-time job. Thandi found it difficult to juggle work and studying, so she stopped studying. She found a full-time job and remits about half her salary to Thoko to help her look after Omphile. Thandi feels that she is not ready to look after Omphile on her own:

> … if something was to happen to my grandmother, I don't think I'm at a point in my life where I am ready to take care of Omphile yet. Financially and mentally I am still trying to grow myself. Bringing her to Johannesburg and raising her – it worries me because I don't know if I can cater for her the ways she is used to now. She literally gets everything

she wants from me and my grandmother … Every day I push so I can be ready.

Thandi sees Omphile every second month. She has made sure that Omphile understands that she has to be away so that in the future she will be better able to take care of her. She explained:

Me and my grandmother keep talking about what if … we actually prepare her for whatever might happen. With me it was different, I didn't know why my mother left me. I didn't know. I found out when I was 18 [years old] that my grandmother was not my real grandmother. They kept a lot of things from me … I want her [Omphile] to know every dynamic of what is going on around her so she doesn't question how anyone feels about her.

In illustrating the transparency in her relationship with her daughter, Thandi centred on understandings of relationships. She said:

Omphile calls my gran 'Mama' and then calls me 'Mommy'. So sometimes she will say things like, 'Thandi, mommy, listen, Mama says that … ' She knows I am her mother. She acknowledges me as her mom but also wants to have the respect to my grandmother because she is … even with me, my grandmother has always been my mom. Like I know the difference between my mom and my grandmother, she knows the difference between me and her grandmother.

Thandi's experience will resonate with many young mothers and echoes experiences in other case studies in this book (see Pillay's case study 3.2). In African communities in South Africa, teenage pregnancy typically engenders anger from parents, teachers, nurses and community members (Bhana et al. 2010; James et al. 2012; Naidoo et al. 2019; Ngabaza 2011). Pregnant teenagers are embarrassed, teased and taunted by their peers, nurses and schoolteachers, and sometimes the general public (Bhana & Mcambi 2013; Mjwara & Maharaj 2018; Shefer et al. 2013). A teenage girl's experience of pregnancy is often lonely, characterised by fear, shame, secrecy and silence, particularly when conception was a result of non-consensual or coerced sex. South Africa has a very high prevalence of coerced sex and gender-based violence. The sexual debut of many young African women occurs in the context of intimate-partner violence or coerced sex (Jewkes 2005; Jewkes et al. 2001; Wood et al. 2007). Most young women report debating the option of termination, but most eventually decide not to undergo abortion for reasons that include religious considerations and moral indictments, but also when their pregnancy is too advanced and it is therefore not a legal option (Pillay et al. 2019).

Since childcare work is gendered (Mkhwanazi et al. 2018; Shefer et al. 2012), young women's female relatives are most likely to step in to care for an infant if the young mother remains in school; if the father's family is involved, his female relatives will care for the child. But until the publication of *Young Families: Gender, Sexuality and Care* (Mkhwanazi & Bhana 2017), the literature on teenage childbearing in South Africa paid little attention to the dynamics of decision-making within families concerning the care of children born to teenaged mothers. While other edited volumes cover the subject of young parents (Morrell et al. 2012; Swartz & Bhana 2009), these publications focus on young fathers or schools, rather than families. In *Young Families*, the contributing authors specifically illustrate the kinds of negotiations that take place by gender and generation regarding who might raise a teenager's child. These chapters disrupt the dominant narrative of pathologising early childbearing, and instead draw attention to the various strategies of families to deal with its occurrence (see specifically Ngabaza & Shefer 2017; Singh & Naicker 2017).

Thandi's narrative is an important challenge to the negative portrayal of teenaged reproduction; it sheds light on the generative aspects of teenaged childbearing. Many young women aspire to have children over and above other educational and employment goals. Those who support these young women are often ignored in accounts of early childbearing, although they are critical in helping young women manage early childbearing and reproduction.

Discourses of risk and vulnerability are used to deter women from early reproduction. In South Africa, as elsewhere, women are having children later in life. However, in the social sciences and humanities literature, little attention had been given to women of 'advanced maternal age' (AMA) – that is, 35 years and older. The omission of their experiences has occurred partly because high rates of teenage pregnancy are linked to the high rates of HIV infection among women aged 15–24, and because of the moral panic around young women's sexual activity.

Contrasting with the previous case study, the case study that follows (2.2) focuses on Nandipha, who became pregnant with her fourth child in her forties. The South African Department of Health (DoH) requires midwives to inform women over the age of 35 about the elevated health risk of stillbirth, preterm birth and foetal abnormalities, and to offer scans and genetic counselling. While some women may think twice about continuing with the pregnancy and seek termination, many women proceed with their pregnancies. Drawing on an interview conducted in 2016 as part of her ongoing research on middle-class African women's experiences of pregnancy and childbirth, Ziyanda Majombozi describes how Nandipha wrestled with the narrative of risk during her pregnancy, and explores the importance of women's interactions with health professionals about 'risky' pregnancies in facilitating hope or hopelessness about the outcome of a pregnancy.

Case study 2.2

Too old to have a baby

Ziyanda Majombozi

Nandipha was 36 weeks pregnant. I was in Cape Town and was able to see her one last time before her baby daughter arrived. I was certain that after having five boys, she would be excited to finally have a girl, and that she was looking forward to the birth. This was not the case. Instead, she said:

> Good thing you are here … I want you to help me with something very important. The nurses have been telling me that I am too old to be pregnant and that anything can happen and that basically, I might die during childbirth. The closer it gets to the time, and the more they keep telling me this, the more worried I become. I need you to help me draft a legal document outlining my wishes for my children should I die. At least I need to know that if I were to die, the boys and hopefully this girl will be taken care of.

I fumbled as I tried to express my anger at how the nurses could keep preaching death at such a life-giving moment, and why they would cause her so much anxiety. Eventually we talked about the idea of drafting a legal document and her wishes, as I recognised that this was a legitimate concern for her and I needed to help her where I could. Not long after our conversation, at 44 years of age, Nandipha gave birth to a beautiful healthy baby girl; they were released from Khayelihle Hospital (pseudonym) in less than a week.

Nandipha's story connects with the broader politics of reproduction. In sub-Saharan Africa and South Asia, one in six women today dies in pregnancy or childbirth. Advanced maternal age accounts for many maternal fatalities. It is associated with increased risk of perinatal and neonatal death, and other pregnancy complications – including preterm delivery, gestational diabetes, pregnancy-induced hypertension, severe pre-eclampsia, anal-sphincter tears, placental abruption, perinatal death, preterm labour, foetal macrosomia, foetal growth restriction, increased Caesarean sections, breech birth, spontaneous abortion and antepartum stillbirth (Jacobsson et al. 2004; Laopaiboon et al. 2014). These risks may inform couples in deciding about pregnancy, and inform policy-makers of the needs in healthcare services for women of advanced maternal age. At the same time, women of advanced maternal age with good general health, and with a chromosomally normal fetus, may have a risk-free delivery and favourable pregnancy outcome (Callaway et al. 2005; Dulitzki et al. 1998). Statistically, pregnancy and birth over the age of 40 are more likely than not to be safe, and perinatal deaths are rare (Jacobsson et al. 2004).

The South African DoH regards pregnancy in women 37 years or older as risky. The department requires midwives to inform these women of the increased risks; and this narrative is the background rhythm in the lives of women like Nandipha as they go about their day-to-day activities. Women who proceed with their pregnancies are often full of anxieties about the possibility of death – their own and that of their child.

Soon after Nandipha's pregnancy was confirmed at the clinic, she was given 'her options'. She was counselled that she would pose risks for herself and her unborn child because of her age. The nurses told her that if her baby survived, she might be deformed and have many illnesses. Nandipha was advised to terminate the pregnancy, but she wanted the baby, regardless, and refused the offer to terminate. She was then asked to sign a document acknowledging that she had been informed of the risks and had chosen to proceed.

Nandipha felt that signing the document gave the nurses permission to instil fear, to abuse her and to ignore her concerns. When I asked her to elaborate, she said:

> Into abayenzayo bayasoyikisa, every time xa ndibuza umbuzo I would
> be told , susisokolisa apha, uthe uyamfuna umntwana wakho noba
> sisdalwa Ubunethuba lo-aborta but awa aborta so noba unexhala lantoni
> ayisokwenza mahluko [What they do is scare us, every time I ask a
> question, I would be told, do not trouble us, you said you want your child
> even if it is deformed. You had the opportunity to abort but you did not.
> Whatever your concern is, it won't make any difference].

Nandipha found these remarks distressing, contributing to feelings of hopelessness and fear that she might lose the baby, her own life or both.

Pregnancies in older age highlight women's sexuality. This contradicted what the nurses believed to be acceptable. Nurses humiliated and abused older women who went to the facility to seek pregnancy-related care. In this way, the nurses policed women's desires to start or expand a family in their late thirties or forties. The nurses talked about how troublesome older women were during labour. Imitating a nurse and slightly raising her voice to mimic shouting, Nandipha said, 'Bathi jonga abantwana bayabeleka quick. Nina nilunywa unyaka onesqhuma. Benihleleleni ningazali nibadala kangaka tana? [They say look, the children (younger women) birth quickly. You (older women) labour forever. What were you waiting for not having children when you are so old?]' One of Nandipha's fears was the abuse older women reported during labour. 'Uphuma ubhonte if uyacotha [You walk out "colourful" if you take long],' said Nandipha, referring to the bruises of older women slapped on their inner thighs by midwives if their labour seemed to take 'too long' or they were not pushing hard enough. Fearful of this, Nandipha asked for an elective Caesarean section. The hospital gynaecologist advised her against this option, saying she was healthy enough for a vaginal birth.

Despite the dominant narratives of risk at the hospital, Nandipha's life outside the hospital continued normally, with day-to-day activities such as taking care of her primary-school-age sons and buying clothes for her new daughter. Nandipha was excited that she would give birth to a beautiful daughter, encouraged by family support and personal prayer. She constantly prayed for a healthy baby and the strength to accept the outcome of the birth. Her sister lived nearby, and Nandipha would call or visit her, frustrated by her treatment in the maternity ward, and would ask for advice: 'Boniswa was a godsend,' Nandipha explained. 'When coming from the clinic, I would go to her and vent about what happened. She would tell me not to worry about what they said, and focus on my baby and staying healthy so that I would have a healthy baby.' Nandipha's other sisters were also looking forward to having a new baby in the family, and outside the abusive hospital space excitement surrounded the pregnancy. This empowered Nandipha, and gave her the strength to continue with the pregnancy and to anticipate a joyous future.

Nandipha's account of pregnancy illustrates the everyday experiences of women of advanced maternal age in public healthcare facilities. Women are commonly abused in public healthcare obstetric units, and nurses are known to humiliate and assert power over patients through shouting, beating and neglect; this is especially so with women who are illiterate or semiliterate (Jewkes et al. 1998). Despite consistent calls to label this 'obstetric violence' (Pickles 2015), nurses continue to mistreat and physically and verbally abuse patients, particularly in townships. Women constantly complained about midwives who were 'rude', 'inhuman' and 'uncaring', who spoke to them with disrespect and without kindness. Over two decades ago, Jewkes et al. (1998) wrote of women's fear of nurses and abuse, meted out to ensure that women behaved 'properly'. Yet still nurses discipline women's bodies and sexuality through fear, humiliation, and violence. Rachel Jewkes et al. (1998) suggest that nurses' abuse creates a 'social distance and maintaining fantasies of identity and power' between them and patients. Some women fight or shout back; others deny the ill treatment, hoping that their silence will minimise the abuse. Nandipha felt that the only way to minimise abuse was to comply, 'to avoid asking many questions, avoid complaining about how the nurses treat you, and making sure that you do not show vulnerability in moments of verbal and sometimes physical abuse.'

Nandipha's experience illustrates the power relations that exist between health practitioners and patients. These mirror broader biopolitics, specifically the politics of reproduction. It also shows us how bodies are regulated in order to produce healthier populations that are successful in their pursuit of meeting national goals – in this example, by eliminating potentially unhealthy children in order to achieve a healthier population (Turner 1992). Medical practices are regulated to suit certain political agendas, and not personal choice and desire. But social norms, and not medical concerns, allow nurses to say *ninezimanga uzala nibadala ngaka* [it is shocking for you to bear children at such an advanced age], speaking to the social unacceptability for women who are 'too old' to reproduce. Faced with narratives of risk, women build spaces where they can go for comfort, spaces where they can gain social support and hope. When determined to expand her family, Nandipha was able to look beyond the abuse at the hospital, and to use her personal networks for support and help to prepare for the arrival of her child.

As a key event in the making of a nation and a country's population, and in benchmarking national health, childbirth is tightly controlled and monitored. Historically, women who were seen as undesirable mothers were sterilised to prevent pregnancy, some without their knowledge (Akyüz et al. 2012; Patel 2017). Today some nurses and doctors police women's reproduction by using a discourse of risk to deter some from having children, and apply punishments to those who continue with a pregnancy despite knowing the risks. Clinics and hospitals are thus involved in policing biological reproduction.

However, a diagnosis of a congenital anomaly prenatally does not necessarily result in a decision to terminate the pregnancy, and women's decisions are not necessarily based on test results or medical advice (Rapp 2000). Various factors influence the choices women make, for example, religious beliefs, financial status, the availability of resources and support, the reproductive experiences of extended family members, and attitudes to disability. Prior experience of a particular disability or disease, medical knowledge, social networks and family situation also play a role in the decision-making. So, too, do local meanings about pregnancy, maternity, prenatal love and adult gender identity (Press & Browner 1994). Further, there is no simple correlation between knowing, meaning and action, and no way to predict how someone will receive the news that their infant is carrying a disease, or has a genetic or other impairment. Even when given information about their child's health, some women may misunderstand what they are being told or reinterpret it in a different way to medical personnel. Women, their partners and their families must navigate the 'gap' created by statistical estimations of risk, their own concerns about taking the test, and their doubts about the meaning of the results (Rapp 2000).

In South Africa, women of 'advanced maternal age' may be offered various tests. These can be liberating, since women are able to know about the health of their foetus. However, tests are not 100 per cent accurate, and a woman may terminate a wanted pregnancy only to be told that the test was a false positive. Some women choose not to take a prenatal diagnostic test because knowing that one may have a child with a disability has major implications in the immediate term for family relationships, and for future decisions. Children with disabilities may need substantial care; some require constant caregiving with associated financial implications. While children with disabilities who require permanent care are eligible for the Care Dependency Grant (valued in April 2019 at R1 780), this amount does not cover the medical and other costs of care. Decisions about whether or not to terminate a wanted pregnancy depend on the cultural background and social circumstances of the person or people making the decisions and on the specific diagnosis. In African communities, there is the added issue of the stigma that often surrounds termination and certain disabilities.

Both private and public maternity-care facilities in South Africa face systemic problems of high national rates of maternal mortality and dramatic increases in maternity-related malpractice suits. In response, increasingly strict, standardised protocols prioritise potential clinical emergency. Some families, when making decisions about care, consider not only immediate clinical risk, but also what they want for future generations. Memories of past humiliations and triumphs, in this generation and in the past, are recalled. Families claiming responsibility for perinatal risk management balance individualised risk assessment in relation to states of mind (such as satisfaction), and values (such as independence and integrity). While case studies 2.1 and 2.2 illustrate how age provokes judgemental responses to women's aspirations to bear children, the following case study (2.3) discusses race as a mediating factor of women's treatment in both public and private hospitals, and the choices that women are given regarding how they give birth and who attends to the birth (see also Andaya 2019; Davis 2019; Quattrocchi 2019). In case study 2.3, Kathleen Lorne McDougall draws on her research conducted in Cape Town between 2014 and 2017 to discuss how considerations of race, history and medical engineering affect the choices that women make about where to give birth and with whom. As in the previous case study, McDougall describes the construction of risk, and how this is used to justify medical interventions.

Case study 2.3

Families, emergency and birth progress after apartheid

Kathleen Lorne McDougall

The timelines on which families base birthing choices are often far longer than those considered by medical professionals as necessary to forestall clinical emergencies. In making birthing choices, the Cape Town families I got to know during my ethnographic fieldwork factored in memories of past humiliations and triumphs in preceding generations. For some families, this was a process that took account of apartheid-era racism. Such multigenerational considerations often took priority over medical concerns regarding clinical risk.

Maternity institutions run by the state are under pressure to reduce maternal mortality rates to meet United Nations Sustainable Development Goals, and private facilities catering for maternity face dramatically rising costs for liability insurance, leading to the practice of legally defensive medicine. The challenges facing state institutions create the sense that private-sector hospitals are sanctuaries, occluding the problem of extremely high rates for Caesarean sections in the private sector. Various pressures to avoid clinical emergency in both the public and private sectors have led to emergency-centric, standardised protocols. Yet, improving perinatal care is not simply a matter of standardising policy according to a global, one-size-fits-all model (Freedman 2016), because there is an idiosyncratic ebb and flow to each labour and familial concern.

Labour progress

Raya felt violated by her three unwanted Caesareans in Cape Town private hospitals: 'With all of them something was taken from me without me wanting it to be taken.' Her first surgery took place at a Cape Town private hospital at 40 weeks, on the grounds that the placenta could be calcifying. Raya discovered later that some calcification at full term is normal. Other common reasons I heard of for scheduled Caesareans were too little amniotic fluid, too big baby or too small pelvis, all diagnoses based on ultrasound scans, difficult to prove but acceptable to medical-insurance companies.

No woman I spoke to was informed of the risks associated with repeat Caesareans, nor informed that a double suture would nullify the small risk of uterine rupture were she to attempt a vaginal birth after the Caesarean. At Raya's third Caesarean, the private-sector doctor quipped that he had sterilised her during the surgery. Raya, furious at the memory, said to me: 'For me having Caesars means that at some point a doctor's going to tell me, "You can't have any more children," and I don't want someone else to make that decision for me.' When she was pregnant for the fourth time in 2015, Raya and her husband, Marcel, selected a home-birth midwife, Margaret, who they were confident could handle slow labour. And, as is likely with any first-time labour and after a Caesarean, Raya's labour did progress slowly. After 30 hours of peaceful labour, with foetal heart rate and Raya's blood pressure monitored with hand-held devices, it looked like Raya was close to giving birth. Margaret looked to see if the baby's head was moving into the vagina, as she expected, and when she couldn't see the head, she checked Raya's cervical dilation. At three centimetres, it was nowhere close to full dilation.

According to the partogram, a graph used in Cape Town hospitals to track cervical dilation, labour should last no longer than 10 hours in total. On the partogram, cervical dilation at a rate of less than one centimetre per hour indicates a potential emergency, even when mother and infant show no signs of distress (for example a decline in foetal heart rate or maternal blood pressure). In general, women in public hospitals are likely to labour, as there is limited capacity for surgery. By contrast, in private hospitals, most patients do not labour, and doctors schedule one or two days a week just to perform Caesareans. As one midwife joked, 'The well-equipped labour wards are so empty that you expect to see tumbleweed rolling along' – as in abandoned frontier towns in classic Westerns.

The high rate of Caesareans in the private sector – at 67 per cent, well over the WHO (World Health Organization) recommendation of 10 per cent – was described to me as a response to the rise in obstetric-related malpractice suits. 'It is easier to defend cutting sooner rather than later,' a Cape Town private obstetrician told me, especially since a Caesarean performed during labour requires more skill than one performed before labour begins. 'A malpractice suit could end a doctor's career,' he continued. Even if a doctor's insurance company covers legal defence, he or she may be unable to get malpractice insurance again.

In public hospitals the approach is driven by perceptions of emergency. Teenagers and foreign-born Africans are especially constrained in how their labours are managed. Tadinawashe, a 17-year-old Zimbabwean first-time mother, received antenatal care from a trained midwife living close to her informal settlement home, and went for a routine antenatal checkup at her local state maternity facility, a midwife-run obstetric unit (MOU). For no stated reason, she was transferred and labour was induced, with the synthetic prostaglandin Misoprostil causing intense uterine contractions. Tadinawashe could not contact her family or midwife. Her cellphone battery needed charging. She could not speak English, Afrikaans or isiXhosa well, and the staff who dealt with her did not speak her home language, Shona. The induced labour did not proceed quickly, and a Caesarean was performed.

I came to know of many cases of obstetric violence in state hospitals (see also Chadwick 2016, 2017). However, many staff worked hard with limited resources to improve women's experiences. An MOU manager painted a vivid picture for me of a midwife or nurse trying to be, as she put it, an octopus in understaffed and overcrowded conditions:

> You are looking after someone, but then someone else comes in screaming that the baby is coming, and you have to leave. And in the background a nurse or a cleaner is shouting that a baby's head is blue and then you have to leave to take care of that situation. It's hectic!

Another MOU manager partnered with an NGO to help midwives debrief after emotional distress and offered a volunteer doula programme for birthing mothers. She sometimes paid for tea and biscuits for recuperating mothers out of her own wages.

Humiliating hospital experiences are not limited to state facilities, nor to birthing, nor are the reasons for avoiding hospitals limited to one generation. For instance, Zainab remembered her father's terminal care for cancer in a state hospital during apartheid, where hospital staff left him lying in his own excrement. As someone classified as 'coloured', he was not allowed to be treated in a whites-only hospital with better-trained staff and better facilities. In this context, Zainab did not wish to use state hospitals for a vaginal birth.

Though agreeing to allow a trial of labour, Zainab's private doctor, previously classified 'white', scheduled her third Caesarean for 39 weeks, one week before the due date. When Zainab asked him to delay the Caesarean until 40 weeks, the doctor became annoyed, and he asked her husband to sign a form absolving him from liability were Zainab to die. Zainab laboured at home for a few days, until, when labour suddenly intensified, she grew scared and rushed to hospital. She arrived there almost fully dilated and still strong in her labour, but to the doctor, the long labour signified emergency. Before examining Zainab, he ordered an epidural so strong she could not speak or open her eyes. He attached a vacuum suction device on the baby's head, forcibly extracting the baby. The vacuum suction cap became detached twice during the procedure. The baby had likely not yet turned into the optimal position to exit the vagina. When the placenta was delivered, Zainab began to bleed internally, and eventually, she was given a hysterectomy to stop the bleeding. Grateful that the surgery saved her life, she did not raise the possibility that the interventions themselves might have caused the bleeding.

Raya, Marcel and Margaret wanted to minimise emergencies like those described above through avoiding emergency-focused care. Margaret's response to Raya's slow labour was, 'This sometimes happens after a Caesarean. The cervix becomes shy, and slow to open up' – making the cervix sound like a vulnerable little creature. Worried that Raya might tire, requiring transfer to hospital for surgery, Margaret asked permission to stretch the cervix open with her fingers – an excruciating procedure, but lasting less than a minute. Raya's cervix was now at eight centimetres, and she birthed her baby a couple of hours later. She and Marcel were triumphant.

The triumph was partly a response to feeling under siege from emergency-focused authorities, an experience that Raya, as a woman of colour, read in racial terms. At Raya's last consultation at the state hospital, the doctor had told her that attempting a vaginal birth after three Caesareans was like running across a busy four-lane freeway. He scheduled a Caesarean for the first available appointment, three days after the consultation. He told Raya this would be her last child, as having another Caesarean was too risky. Later Marcel checked out the doctor's Facebook page, and found triumphant posts each time the surgeon (a young white man) sterilised a woman (usually African). The doctor was worried about overpopulation and poverty, and Raya and Marcel now questioned his motives.

Marcel and Raya associated vaginal birth with family responsibility, and their fiercely held autonomy. This stance was a powerful contrast to the historical backdrop of apartheid-style totalitarianism. Although Raya could not remember racial segregation – she was born only two years before the first democratic South African elections – her parents, classified as 'coloured', could, although they did not talk about it. Raya remembered her grandmother telling her of giving birth to three children vaginally, two at home, after a Caesarean section. Her grandmother's waters broke a week before she gave birth: this would now be a sign for intervention for fear of infection. Raya's grandmother had an enviable freedom of choice over birthing. Raya told me that she hated how doctors put unreasonable fear in women.

Clinical/social emergency

Doctors' concerns specifically regard clinical events – for example prolonged labour, uterine rupture, haemorrhage – as in need of surgical intervention and episiotomies. These are distinct from fear of spiritual defilement (Wikan 2013). If labour is considered purely as physiological event, then interventions, even if seen by women as humiliating or violating, are considered ethical if necessary to forestall an emergency. As Peter Redfield (2016) argues, medical emergency is conceptually associated with exceptional moments, marked by definitive action, that exclude non-medical considerations (including systemic political ones). Although speedy surgical action may be essential to save a mother's or infant's life, the cases I became interested in were the unexceptional majority, where risky pharmaceutical and surgical interventions, to induce or speed up labour or to deliver via Caesarean, were defined by protocols to safeguard against emergencies.

Any medical happening is a matter of signification, of reading symptoms, trying to predict their outcome, and making sense of what is manifest. In a medical emergency, what is treated is to some extent always a probability, even just a possibility. Treatment affects outcome, and it is never certain what might have happened had there been no intervention or what might have transpired in the absence of clinical facilities. Institutional processes and fear of hospital settings are likely both to slow labour and, in a 'fear cascade' (Stenglin & Foureur 2013), to cause additional invasive interventions to prevent catastrophe.

What is understood as catastrophic or beneficial in birthing has come to be expressed in terms of averages and risk probabilities, but also to be highly medicalised. While medicalised birthing may be essential, it replicates humiliations associated with colonial and apartheid medical care. Further, in South Africa and elsewhere, particularly on the African continent, maternal mortality rates reflect deep systemic social inequality, so that policy shifts towards standardised institutional care to reduce maternal mortality rates may also seem to heal deep systemic social inequality. However, increasingly medicalised birthing procedures are historically and pragmatically entangled with racialised inequality (see also Andaya 2019; Davis 2019; Quattrocchi 2019).

Southern African birth and modern progress

Cervical dilation was first correlated with length of labour in Emanuel Friedman's 1950s study in New York City (see Cohen & Friedman 2018). Friedman sought a physical point of comparison for different labour experiences. He suggested an average and so normal (and abnormal) lengths of labour. In the work of southern Africa-based obstetrician R.W. Philpott, the partogram came to be associated with *both* clinical protocol and social development. Philpott, working in then Rhodesia (now Zimbabwe) added an alert and an action line to Friedman's graph. The lines indicated when, during labour, midwives in poorly equipped satellite clinics should prepare to transfer patients to base hospitals with surgeons, theatres and blood supplies. The partogram became important in South Africa when, in the 1970s, midwife-run obstetric units were being established in Cape Town to extend allopathic maternity care to women of colour.

Philpott (1978: 833) argued that his partogram would enable every woman to have a medicalised delivery, as was fundamental to modern progress. Although framed simply to support social empowerment and alleviate poverty through access to medical care, the partogram was bound up with the political emergency of the time. The 1970s in Rhodesia were marked by violent civil action against Ian Smith's racist regime; in South Africa, the Afrikaner Nationalist police and defence force responded violently to civil protests. Civil rights were increasingly suspended through successive states of emergency in the 1980s. In this period, a high rate of African fertility was considered an emergency not because of rising poor populations, but because of fears that the African population in South Africa might further outnumber the white population. A system of fertility control for African women was put in place, and by 1976 birth centres and fertility control programmes increased. By providing birthing facilities in neighbourhoods for people of colour, women need not give birth in hospitals in areas designated for those classified as white. Families were disciplined by racial boundaries.

At time of writing, 40 years later, birthing possibilities, fertility control, emergency and race continue to be entangled. The extension of hospital care to African populations also extended regulatory control over birth. Relations with doctors and nurses continue to be inflected by race, interpreted by those involved as part of a racialised or nationalised story – as Raya and Marcel understood limiting their fertility, and as Tadinawashe understood her experience in relation to xenophobia. Medical emergency, as defined for birthing women, continues to be conflated with various social, political, historical and economic emergencies, and efforts to avoid emergencies are enacted on women's bodies. Further, in an emergency-focused paradigm, not of civil unrest but of globalised Millennium Development Goals and now Sustainable Development Goals, maternal mortality rates (MMRs) have become economically and politically very significant.

For low- and middle-income countries (LMICs) like South Africa, perceptions of political instability result in lowered international credit ratings and reduced economic potential, affecting not only the private sector but also state investment funds. Images of hospital horrors conjure spectres of state infrastructural collapse, reinvigorating a modernist imaginary of horrifying savagery run rampant. In this context, South Africa's 2013 MMR of 141 per 100 000 deaths, triple the United Nations goal for 2015, suggests a lack of economic and social progress, as illustrated by a *Mail & Guardian* headline: 'Birth a measure of progress: Reducing maternal and newborn mortality has to be a priority if Africa is to reach its potential' (25 January 2013). However, if reducing the MMR and insurance liability involves increasing interventions, women are stripped of autonomy, affecting families of all races and echoing apartheid-era race-based fertility humiliation. Increased medical interventions subjugate women to doctors and nurses. Paradoxically, the intent to save lives in these particular ways makes it difficult for families to find ways of redressing racialised birth-related humiliations.

In 2017 Raya had her fifth child with a vaginal birth at home. The month before birth, she saw a doctor as a precautionary measure, and he wanted to deliver by Caesarean. Raya resisted again. As is typical of second-time vaginal births, labour was much shorter – this time only four hours – and the birth was uncomplicated.

For centuries women have given birth at home, with the support of other women – midwives. However, from the early twentieth century, with concern about extremely high infant and maternal mortality rates, childbirth shifted from the home to the hospital, and from the care of midwives (mostly women) to general practitioners and obstetricians (largely men). As pregnancy and childbirth were increasingly medicalised, there was less reliance on women's embodied knowledge (Davis-Floyd 1992; Press & Browner 1994), and medical technologies were used routinely. Pharmaceutical and surgical interventions became increasingly common to manage previously expected or accepted experiences of pregnancy: thalidomide, for instance, was prescribed in the 1960s for nausea in pregnancy, resulting in more than 1 000 children in 46 countries being born with birth defects. In South Africa thalidomide was often combined with other drugs to reduce the risk of side effects, and while there were no reports of birth defects, an increasing number of people suspect that their disability was related to thalidomide (Julie Parle, pers. comm.).

In the 1960s and 1970s, women in Europe and North America became increasingly vocal about their reproductive rights, including when to have children, the right to contraception, where to give birth, and who to attend the birth. Home birthing activists and midwives argued that giving birth in hospitals was not optimal for the mother and child, although they also recognised that for some women, medical interventions were life-saving (Kline 2019). In South Africa, the natural childbirth movement gained strength in the 1990s, and white, middle-class women increasingly chose to give birth at home, with midwifery support, or at birthing centres with access to hospital technologies; such centres were initially available primarily to these women (Chadwick & Foster 2012). For *all* middle-class women who choose to have natural childbirth, the cost of giving birth at home with a midwife or in a private birth clinic is cheaper than an emergency Caesarean and the recovery days spent in a private hospital. They are also less likely to be subjected to interventions, whether these are scheduled, because the woman or the foetus is deemed 'at risk', or are conducted as an emergency measure, when the woman's or the infant's life is threatened.

African women, especially in rural areas, had given birth at home with local midwives or community nurses for generations; for them, access to hospitals and their life-saving technologies was welcome. During apartheid, a two-tier health system operated, providing white South Africans with access to services equivalent to those available in industrialised countries; for all other racial groups medical services at hospitals and clinics were basic (Coovadia et al. 2009). Rural South African women often had to travel great distances to reach a clinic, waiting in long queues to see medical personnel. Post-apartheid, there have been attempts to address the health disparities, but cost remains an obstacle for poor South Africans. Their only options are government local clinics and public hospitals that are chronically under-resourced.

In the next case study (2.4), Cheyenne Jordaan examines a young, white, middle-class couple's ideal birthing aspirations. Jordaan conducted ethnographic research in Johannesburg on the experiences of women and midwives at a private birth centre in 2017. She describes Daniela's and Marco's expectations and fears regarding the imminent birth of their first child. As they describe a recent visit to the obstetrician–gynaecologist (whom they refer to simply as 'the gynae') and the possible outcomes of the pregnancy, they reflect on the meanings of becoming a family, on parenting roles, on intimacy, and on the support from their respective families. They illustrate the nuances and uncertainties around pregnancy and childbirth, and how birthing includes the moment of childbirth and beyond.

Case study 2.4

Birthing Lessy

Cheyenne Jordaan

Daniela and Marco, a couple I spent time with on Monday evenings at antenatal classes, agreed to meet me for coffee. I walked through the glass doors into an atmosphere of freshly ground coffee and the chatter of patrons, and joined them in a corner. Marco ordered me a cappuccino as Daniela began to tell me about her day.

Critical advice, medical risk

They had just come from Daniela's 34-week scan, and so our conversation began with this:

> Today has made me anxious. I have always had this fear of going to a gynae [obstetrician–gynaecologist] who was only going to pressurise me for a C-section [Caesarean section] because it is convenient. Today we found out that she might be away over our due date. I thought, is there a possibility of induced labour? I want to carry to full term but I told her I was willing to bring the date forward. She agreed to let me try an induction as long as I give birth within the 24 hours.

Marco's food arrived. He ate while Daniela continued to explain, with scepticism, her gynae's concerns about the size of her baby's head:

> She was saying the head size is almost two weeks ahead of time, worrying that baby's head is not going to fit in the pelvis. She has booked me in three weeks' time to see. For now, the baby's head is down, but she is going to give me time to allow for the baby to drop more.

After spending some time in midwife Judy's antenatal classes, Daniela had become critical about these suggestions: 'I have this negativity because I am almost trying to block the C-section. I am questioning everything. Had we not gone to Judy's classes, we would not have known if she was speaking the truth or not.' Marco nodded. Daniela paused to sip on her coffee.

'During my scan, she pointed out the calcification of the placenta,' she continued. 'She even asked me if I was a smoker. I told her I'm not.' Daniela recalled the function of the placenta from Judy's classes. A calcifying placenta could place her baby in danger. 'I remembered what Judy had said. If the placenta is affecting the baby and if the baby is better outside than inside, then that's the way we need to go.' Daniela worried about the increasing risks in what had been an uncomplicated pregnancy. The couple gathered information from their antenatal classes, the Web and other media, about risk and the scans. Sometimes this information was overwhelming: 'I had this information overload and I switched off. All the 'ifs' made me question [the doctor's] intentions. I am just anxious about everything now.'

Imagining becoming a family

Daniela and Marco had planned for a natural birth at a private hospital:

> I imagine going to Southville Hospital. They have a new labour ward. I need to know if I am in early stage labour, you know, if it is just Braxton Hicks [contractions] or proper labour. Both my doctor and midwife have explained it to us. I think I have a pretty good idea … The plan would be to just go in and assess how far I am and go from there.

Marco had attended all the antenatal classes, and found them useful in providing preparation for and insight into the possibilities: 'Once we get there, we hope to be guided. We are first-timers, so we are not quite sure. We can imagine but most of it comes from what we have learned in the antenatal classes. We have that guideline. I mean they are the professionals; they do this every day.'

Judy's antenatal classes shaped their expectations and gave Daniela a sense of agency in her pregnancy, helping her to feel prepared. 'Had we not gone to Judy, I would be completely clueless. Whatever they say I would do and not have any opinion on it. It has definitely helped us. I know what to expect even though I have never experienced it … I do not like surprises,' Daniela said with a soft laugh. They understood birth to be unpredictable. Marco explained the importance of information about childbirth: 'It's worse not knowing, the fear of the unknown. I think the Caesar is more organised – on this day at this time – natural birth is like you are waiting for something to happen.'

Daniela continued to explain that her 'gynae' had admitted that a C-section was more controlled: 'You know the history, you know the background, you do this procedure … I might have had a perfect pregnancy but in the last week have complications.' Marco added, 'As we saw from the class … many things can prevent you from having a normal birth, and it was important for us to know … We are the type of people that like to know what we are getting into. We like being organised.' Even so, Marco and Daniela were reluctant to consider surgery outright.

The 'normal' as the natural

Midwife Judy referred to natural birth as 'normal' birth. Daniela explained this as follows:

> I think it depends on your choice. I feel strongly about natural birth. The way I understand this is that previously there wasn't any choice, so why do we have that choice today? Why are women chickening out of the natural birth? Is it really easier? Is it because it's less painful?

Marco associated the term 'normal birth' with natural birth:

> When I hear the word 'normal', I think natural, or how it was intended to be. I mean, look at animals. That is how they do it, and that's how we should be having babies … A Caesarean is a major surgery. Major surgery is not normal to me. I think it should only be done if there is a good reason behind it.

Natural birth here is described as the norm; Caesarean section is spoken of as 'the other birth.' The couple agreed that natural birth was normal birth, and despite their comments about 'not liking surprises', which might have favoured a C-section, their birth plan focused on natural delivery.

Daniela mentioned that she and Marco were regularly asked about their birth choice. Referring to another couple, Daniela remarked,

> When I tell people that I'm having natural birth, they ask 'Why do you want to do that to yourself?' They start with 'Did you know …' The did-you-knows aren't going to change my mind. I get questions like 'Are you going to push this child out? Have you seen the size of this child?' They tell me my body will never be the same again afterward.

Intimacy after childbirth

The conversation shifted to stories about intimacy after childbirth: 'The aunts, uncles, and friends tell us that we have other options. They tell us how my body is going to change, especially down there,' said Daniela. Marco smiled awkwardly. We began discussing stories about how natural birth might impact on intimacy and sexual activities.

'It is the physical part of what birth does to your body,' Daniela explained. 'My cousins are all boys and they often joke around with Marco that it's never going to be the same again and that it's never going to feel the same.' Marco interjected, sounding irritated, 'Maybe if it was from someone who has actually experienced it, I'll take their advice, but people who are saying it are men who have never actually had children.' Daniela added, 'It is not like the intimacy part is never going to work again. If that was the case no one would ever have more than one child.' Part of becoming a family is a reshaping of intimate and sexual engagements.

Pain management

Daniela's discussion of pain management was embedded in the narratives of birth she had gathered from personal networks:

> When you are adamant for natural [birth] they ask, 'Are you going to have an epidural?' Their whole perspective is, if you're having natural birth and you're not going to feel the pain, you might as well have a Caesar. I am still going to push this child out, feeling 90 per cent of the pain or 40 per cent of the pain. They are not going to cut me open so that I can avoid the pain. If I am at that point where I need an epidural, then I will make the call. I will probably decide on the day, if I really needed it …

Marco added his support: 'If it is needed, then it's a good thing. As long as there are no side effects or anything that could harm her or the baby. I am cool with it.'

Family expectations and support systems

Part of the couple's pregnancy journey involved support and expectations of others. Daniela spoke about her relationship with her mother, who had been a nurse in a labour ward and had assisted with deliveries:

> She understands C-sections need to be done sometimes. But, she also knows that obstetricians are very quick to push for C-sections unnecessarily. She is happy to let us make up our own minds … My dad is very old school. I think he likes the idea that we are wanting to go with a natural birth.

Marco continued:

> My parents have not said much about our decision. They don't really make recommendations. We tell them what we want and they are supportive either way. My brother and his wife had two elective Caesars. My mom had a Caesar and Daniela's mom had natural. Our close family have been very supportive of our decisions.

With their parents' support, Daniela and Marco were able to wade through the conflicting advice without feeling unsettled. Becoming a family moved beyond Daniela and Marco as a unit. It involved an exchange of thoughts, advice, guidance and stories. This support would be paramount.

Lessy's birth

I walked through the sliding glass doors of Southville Hospital (pseudonym), making my way through the passages and stairways to meet Daniela and Marco. Marco had been admitted after complications with his recent abdominal surgery, but they had both agreed to meet with me in the coffee shop in the hospital foyer. They were excited to tell me all about the birth of their daughter a few months earlier. We met in the surgery ward, and once Marco was free of the drip and able to leave the ward, we went to the coffee shop in the foyer, buzzing with people, visitors, and patients. We ordered our coffees and Daniela's snack, and chatted about Lessy. Daniela showed me photographs of Lessy from the day she was born. I smiled, now able to put a face to the tiny being. Marco told me how fast she had grown. Daniela described her birth as a wonderful experience. This was despite the three failed inductions in an attempt to initiate labour at 37 weeks. After her failed inductions, a Caesarean section followed. Marco told me that they were grateful that they had had the C-section:

> Some things are meant to be. When Lessy came out, the cord was wrapped around her neck twice. I didn't know until afterward, when the doctor had told me that if Daniela had delivered naturally, it could have been a disaster. It would have strangled [Lessy]. I actually watched the film [of the birth] again, and saw the nurse pulling the cord over Lessy's head. In that moment I did not notice, you know, I was just so excited to meet her.

Achieving what they had previously regarded as a 'normal birth' no longer mattered. The couple were thrilled that Lessy and Daniela were healthy.

The couple had decided not to know the baby's biological sex until birth. Marco said, 'I knew she was a little girl when the gynae held her up and said, "Here she is." Daniela began to tell me about their family members who had been waiting at the hospital in anticipation. She explained that Marco had instructed the gynae 'not to give anything away' when Daniela exited the theatre. Daniela laughed as she told the story:

> Our family hounded her [the gynae] about whether it was a boy or a girl.
> They were just so excited! But we held out; they were getting so mad.
> Eventually, Marco sent a group message saying 'Welcome, Lessy Santos'.
> We could hear them all the way from my room, going crazy.

The support that had been present throughout their pregnancy filled the maternity ward with excitement and love in welcoming their new family member, and this – not the Caesarean section – was paramount to Marco's and Daniela's positive experience in the hospital.

Marco smiled warmly at the memory of Lessy's birth. It was, he said, one of the most memorable moments of his life. Daniela recounted her experience in theatre:

> It was quite strange, you can feel them tugging at you, but you feel no pain.
> I couldn't move my legs at all. They had put up a sheet so that I couldn't
> see them cutting me. What was scary was I began to black out at one stage.
> You actually won't believe how quickly they get that baby out.

I asked Daniela if the videos from the classes had helped her prepare for the spinal block. 'Look, once you are in theatre, the doctors kind of take over,' she said. 'It was surreal. I don't think anything can really prepare you.'

Marco began to talk about his daughter:

> The hardest part about being here is that I was not initially allowed to see
> Lessy. She couldn't come into the ward. Daniela had found the window of
> my room from the outside and I could see her like that. It broke my heart.
> I even gave her little kisses through the glass. I miss her.

'She just cried and cried,' Daniela lamented. Then the couple spoke about the adjustment of becoming parents. Daniela said,

> Marco had lost his job in the last few weeks of our pregnancy. It was
> unimaginably stressful knowing we were about to have a little one and that
> there was going to be no money to support her. We would not have made
> it if we did not have the support of our families. Thankfully, he found a job
> the week I was to be induced. The relief … it was then that we realised our
> priorities as a couple had fundamentally changed. Our focus became Lessy.

Lessy had become the centre of their lives, plans, and relationship. They told me about their love for strict routine in keeping Lessy's daily activities in check, so that they could schedule time for themselves in the early evening. Having a baby changed their life, their relationship and their priorities.

With an increased number of websites explaining medical conditions and procedures, as well as chatrooms for people who have been patients, women now have many ways of getting information on pregnancy and childbirth. However, first-time mothers, even if they feel empowered to question what they are told, must also place their trust in their attending obstetricians, whose 'authoritative knowledge' (Jordan 1978) on childbirth derives from their specialist scientific knowledge and its evidence and technologies.

In case study 2.4, although Daniela and Marco had planned for a natural birth, in the end Lessy was delivered by Caesarean section because Daniela's obstetrician would be on holiday when the baby was due to be born. Even so, the couple managed to rewrite their birth experience as 'wonderful' and 'memorable', because of their families' excitement and support of the birth of their first baby.

The earlier case studies in this chapter also touched on the importance of emotional and/or financial support from families, for first and for subsequent births. For decades, migrant workers have been attracted to Johannesburg – the economic capital and most populous city in South Africa – from elsewhere in South Africa and beyond. Finding housing and employment in the city is not easy, particularly for migrants without legal documentation. For those with documentation, and for internal migrants, building and maintaining social networks and familial ties is key to survival. Soweto – the South Western Townships of Johannesburg – attracts people from throughout South Africa and beyond in search of work and a better life. It is also home to the largest public health hospital – Chris Hani Baragwanath Hospital. Soweto is the backdrop of a number of our case studies which focus on different aspects of everyday life there (see Jewett Nieuwoudt's case study 3.1 and Huschke's case study 3.4).

Poverty and HIV mould quality of life, as men and women juggle low-paid jobs and periods of dependency on friends and family members. Not all women have access to emotional or financial support, and this can make their experiences of pregnancy and motherhood difficult. In case study 2.5, Langelihle Mlotshwa and Sonja Merten draw on their research conducted in Soweto from 2015 to 2019, and describe how single women there negotiate their prospects of becoming mothers, and how this reshapes the meaning of family. As case study 2.5 illustrates, migrant women from Mozambique, Zimbabwe, Lesotho, Swaziland and other parts of southern Africa must negotiate pregnancy, risk of HIV, and the future (Collinson et al. 2007; Walker 2017).

Case study 2.5

Single in Soweto

Langelihle Mlotshwa and Sonja Merten

Despite the fluidity of relationships that has occurred with other changes in South Africa in recent decades, families continue to be often the central pillar of people's lives in terms of economic, social, and emotional support (Mlotshwa et al. 2017). The fluidity of relations leads to ad hoc modalities of social support, to unstable partnerships, sexual relations and intimacy. In this case study, we focus on how single pregnant women negotiate intimate relationships, and family relations of the baby to be born, and access material and emotional support for themselves and their child.

Robyn

Robyn had finished high school in a town in the Northern Cape, and then moved, at age 17, to live with her uncle in Johannesburg, where she started working in a bank while studying business administration. Soon after she moved she became pregnant; her first son was now eight years old. The relationship with the child's father had not lasted, and at the same time she also lost her parents.

When we first met, Robyn was 20 weeks pregnant from a new man, David, but that relationship had faltered. Although David still ran errands for her, she insisted they were not together – he had had other partners concurrently, and Robyn felt emotionally abused. Robyn found herself constantly stressed and depressed; she was admitted to hospital, when she discovered she was pregnant. Her depression deteriorated, and she became suicidal. She was diagnosed with bipolar disorder, started treatment and went for counselling; there she was advised to keep her distance from the father of her child and concentrate on getting better. She tearfully explained that David had wanted her to abort because he was not ready for another child; he had just had another child with a former girlfriend.

Once the baby was born, however, David would take Robyn and the child to hospital or a community clinic. Robyn hoped that David would contribute financially to raising their child out of his own will, but while he was interested in resuming his relationship with Robyn, he seemed less interested in the child. She finally took David to court for maintenance, as she anticipated she would have to raise the child alone. But she also thought that because the child was a boy, he would later want to look for his father for guidance into adulthood, maybe for inheritance, or a sense of identity.

About 11 months after giving birth, Robyn found another boyfriend, who provided emotional support to her and her baby. He was married. Then his wife died, and their relationship also began to deteriorate, and Robyn decided to keep her distance from him as well. She turned to her friends for support and comfort. They took her to church and spent time with her, to distract her from worrying about the relationship. Robyn felt that if her parents were still alive, things would have been better.

Khethiwe

Khethiwe moved to South Africa because of economic hardship in Zimbabwe. She had lived in rural Zimbabwe as a child, then moved to an urban area to start working as a maid. She and her friends decided they could move to South Africa, and in Johannesburg she moved in with her friend.

Khethiwe needed to work to take care of her relatives back home. She worked first as a maid, then in a hotel. But late nights of work took a toll on her health and, without a car to travel at night, she finally left. For some time her family in Johannesburg looked after her, as she could not pay for her accommodation and utilities. When we met her, she had found employment again as a maid, and was happy enough.

She had had three boyfriends before her current boyfriend, and had tried to get pregnant to no avail. After four miscarriages, she felt unloved and unwanted, desperate that she might never have children: the men had all left her because of the miscarriages. Then she met a new man, already married, and he supported her while she was unemployed. After some time, she explained, they fell in love and started sleeping together without condoms; a few months later she was pregnant. She was fearful she would lose the child. Khethiwe felt that she 'deserved' this man; he was loving and just 'perfect'. She accepted that they had to hide their relationship from his wife and church members. She hoped that one day he might make her his second wife. But she was happy that he was providing and caring for her. However, she also said that if another man came in her life, and accepted and loved her, then she would leave the relationship she was in.

There was one unresolved problem. When Khethiwe was pregnant, she discovered that she was HIV positive. She asked herself how she could tell her boyfriend, whether she had given him HIV, and whether his wife was infected. What would happen to her, and who would help? At the time of the last interview, she still hadn't disclosed her HIV status to her partner.

The absence of natal family members makes pregnancy without a partner difficult. Many migrants struggle with acceptance from the receiving community, and feel vulnerable (Grove & Zwi 2006; Lori & Boyle 2015). In these circumstances, women reshape and invent new forms of relationships, and, as illustrated in case study 2.5, may be willing to establish relationships with married men or have unplanned children as a way to secure a relationship. Pregnant women find ways to survive, with or without a formal family arrangement, to make their lives better, to protect themselves and their children (see Huschke's case study 3.4). As long as a man provides emotional and material support, women may be happy with the relationship – at least in the short term.

Robyn and Khetiwe both migrated to Johannesburg for work and a better life. Robyn was an internal migrant, and in Johannesburg lived with her uncle; Khetiwe knew only the friends with whom she had travelled from Zimbabwe. Educated and South African, Robyn had a better chance of finding employment than Khetiwe, for whom the city was likely a lonely experience, with xenophobic attitudes limiting her employment opportunities and use of government services. As Deirdre Blackie (2017) notes in her study on child abandonment in South Africa, the loss of family support during pregnancy is critical to women's decisions to keep or abandon their child at birth. Migrant women without papers are especially vulnerable. Migrant women may be rejected by their natal families, and cannot apply for child maintenance from reluctant boyfriends. Further, without papers proving their residential status, they are unable to legally give their child up for adoption. While many women do not abandon their child, abandonment is reported to be on the rise.[1] As Blackie argues, abandonment reflects the 'desperation and isolation' of women for whom psychological, legal and economic factors make the idea of raising a child virtually impossible (2017: 203; see also case study 3.3).

The case studies presented so far all relate to children born of heterosexual relationships, and reflect heterosexual ideals of family and parenthood. In the final case study of this chapter (2.6), Casey Golomski and Gabby Dlamini consider the reproductive and parenting aspirations of gay, lesbian, transgender, intersex, asexual, or queer members of a grassroots Pentecostal Christian Church. Their research was conducted in township communities outside Mbombela and involved in-depth interviews from May to June 2017. For those whose sexual orientation was not accepted by their families, church membership strengthened the sense of worth of these individuals. A few had been coerced by their families into heterosexual relationships or marriage, and some had children from these relationships. But most were unmarried, with same-sex partners, and desired to have children. Same-sex, opposite-gender partners anticipated having children by assisted reproductive technologies or adoption, and desired to be caring and domestically and financially supportive parents for their children, who would be their 'beautiful blessings'.

Case study 2.6

Beautiful blessings

Casey Golomski and Gabby Dlamini

What kinds of parents do South African gay men and lesbians want to be? What reproductive and parental decision-making challenges do they face in their families and communities? In this case study, we focus on the reproductive and parenting aspirations of members of a grassroots South African Pentecostal Christian church called Ark of Joy, based primarily in Mpumalanga and Gauteng provinces. Ark of Joy does not claim to be a 'gay church', but nearly all members identify as lesbian, gay, bisexual, transgender, intersex, queer, or asexual (which, following our interlocutors, we abbreviate to LGBTIQA). The church is known for an ethos of inclusivity and support for people across spectrums of gender and sexuality. Church leaders and members are also well integrated in activist and health-research networks.

Currently LGBTIQA persons' rights and freedom from discrimination based on sexual orientation are protected by the South African Constitution. Still, many LGBTIQA South Africans live discretely: they do not feel 'open' or 'free' to express their sexual identities. They refer to themselves and each other as 'after 9'; that is, they feel free only after dark to send messages to, call or meet romantic partners, or dress in opposite-gender clothing. Verbal and structural discrimination against sexual minorities are common; violence against lesbians especially is a terrible reality in some communities.

Raised and living in postcolonial, predominantly Christian communities in South Africa, many LGBTIQA people have deeply personal and familial relationships with Christianity. It is no surprise then to find a small but rich community of gay and lesbian Christians. A few urban gay and lesbian churches in South Africa are globally connected, but Ark of Joy is a grassroots organisation. The globalisation of Pentecostal–charismatic Christianity is driving cultural and religious innovation, and Ark of Joy adopts this kind of sensational aesthetics of prayer healing, speaking in tongues, and focus on the Holy Spirit.

Ark of Joy was founded in 2007 after a few activist gay men and lesbians, including several pastors, decided to organise a church catering to LGBTIQA community needs. The church first organised in the township of Nelspruit (renamed Mbombela in 2009), and this inspired new branches to be formed in the region. The church in 2019 has around 400 congregants and regularly hosts interchurch gatherings at Easter and on other holidays, as well as educational and spiritual workshops. Within the church, members may affiliate to one of three committees: the youth committee, the 'men's committee', and *idwala*, meaning the 'stone' or 'foundation'.

Our 32 case-study participants largely configured their sex–gender identities in binary form. In interviews, they identified as either men/males (M) or women/females (F): 21 self-identified as female (ages 18–42, mean 19 years), and 11 as male (ages 18–42, mean 25 years). Of the 18 self-identified females who identified as lesbian, 10 variably said they were 'femme' or 'feminine', and 8 were 'masculine' or 'butch'. Of the remaining 3, 1 identified as asexual, one as bisexual, and 1 as transgender. All males identified as gay: 7 as 'femme' or 'more like a woman', and 4 as 'masculine'. Many respondents also noted an individual self in their answers:

'I am just me.' They repeatedly highlighted these sex–gender binaries, which then framed views on reproduction choices and relationship roles.

Having children, changing oneself

Four participants (2 M, 2 F) had biological children; only 1, a lesbian, had her child, a 12-year-old girl, living with her. Most participants who did not have children wanted them in the present or the foreseeable future. Some saw themselves as unprepared economically, emotionally and socially: 'I do not have kids but I want some … Kids are a blessing from God. I believe I must have one … but there is monetary pressure due to how expensive they are. We should plan' (Priscilla, 39); 'I want children maybe when I'm 40. For now, I'm focusing on building myself up. I do want something to leave behind, so eventually, yes' (Mlandvo, 20); 'A home without a child is boring. At least with a [future] child, I would know that I would have a child to support. I would like to [in the future] say "I have a child" ' (Lerato, 19).

Lerato's statement about life being 'boring' was not about immaturity or being 'supported' as a teenage girl who looks forward to relying on others after becoming pregnant. Rather, it reflects the need to have a child as part of a life trajectory and a rite of passage. Several men and women discussed having children as part of a new life stage or an obvious part of the progression of life. The rhetoric of descent and continuity was also both socially and individually transformative: 'Children are the next generation of my family. I am what I am because of them' (Bontle, 19); 'I want two children. I think the fact that they are so young and innocent, that I can give someone the opportunities that I didn't. That I can correct my wrongs through that person. I can be a better person to that child than my parents [were to me]' (Kevin, 29).

Excepting Kevin, nearly all participants said they grew up happily and had good childhood experiences. Most reported that their families were loving and supportive, and more than half still lived with mothers, grandmothers, or another relative. A few experienced intolerance, but they more often felt discrimination in the broader community or in churches other than Ark of Joy.

Care, love, and support: Being good, gendered parents

We asked participants what kind of person they would want to have children with or what made a good parent. People commonly spoke about love, care, support, and the provision of housing, food and clothing. A good parent was one who would provide for children and the household. Answers often reflected participants' own sexual and gender identities, and idealised gender roles of caregiving and providing. A few participants joked that a same-sex partnership could have, for example, 'two moms,' but more often participants qualified what this meant. Kealaboga (24) identified her future child's ideal parent as follows:

> [She would be] lesbian, obviously. It's a matter of having someone who
> we can raise the child with. Somebody who's full of love. Who believes in
> herself. Someone who understands that things do not always happen the
> way they want them to. Someone who will be a mom to my kids. Who will
> protect them. Not a second dad, another mom.

Kealaboga self-identified as lesbian – 'I was so gay' growing up, she reported, laughing, but she did not identify as masculine nor consider herself a male in the relationship. She stated her lesbian partner would not be 'another dad', but would adopt the 'mom' role. For most participants, to be 'feminine' most often included material components like make-up, clothing, and other 'girly' things. Some, though, emphasised self-respect, independence and the capacity to love children as constitutive of being feminine. Being feminine was not about being female, however. A young masculine gay man said:

> I don't base a woman on their biological gender, but on the gender which
> they feel they belong to. It means having a feminine side separate from a
> macho side. [A feminine person] takes care of the kids. They feed them.
> They don't have to bear the children to be a woman. Just taking care of
> someone is what it means to be a woman (Pule, 18).

What it meant to be a man or woman differed from femininity (if we asked about being a woman), or masculinity (when we asked about being a man). Sometimes participants said they were the same thing. Still, for those who differentiated these gender-presentation categories, heteronormative roles were at play. To be masculine was associated with being a 'breadwinner' or financial provider of the family, or being more reserved or assertive. A masculine person was someone who needed to be given respect and status by others who depended on him or her: '[To be masculine is] to provide and care for the family. To be the breadwinner. To show love if you have family' (Thuso, 21); 'It means to be more of a man. To be physically strong. To be strong for your family. A woman can be masculine, but I do not feel that it is necessary. It means to be a husband, a father, and to be strong for your family' (Tlali, 25).

Of course, finding 'the perfect' man or woman to be a parent for one's future children was challenging: 'If only that [person] existed,' one self-identified 'butch' lesbian told us, 'someone who is full of tender love and care, someone with a sense of humour, someone who is religious, someone like me' (Vanessa, 25). Overall, love, care and financial capacity to provide were the dominant qualities of a good parent, regardless of sexual orientation or gender identity and role in the relationship. One participant, an effeminate gay man, summed this up in a way that revealed the precarity of living and raising children in township communities:

> Yes, I wish to have kids. But to have kids, I would be their mother. We would not go to a sperm donor. They would have their father and they would call me mom. My partner would have to respect me before we have kids; there must be good communication between us. Must work, handsome, love himself, must not get drunk. If we do drink, we must at least maybe get drinks and drink from home because then we will be planning and building our future, our home. He must not hit the kids. If the child needs something they must be able to get it and not see it only at their friends and not always told, 'It will come, it will come.' For example, if the child wants a dictionary from school we can buy it. (Sello, 26)

Acquiring children: Sperm and perils of adoption

Same-sex relationships required thoughtful planning to acquire desired children. Participants ranged from accepting their partners' existing children to wanting to adopt or to undertake assisted reproduction. 'Sperm' and artificial insemination were often mentioned; the term 'sperm donation' included going to surrogates and in reference to a male partner in a relationship: 'We may consult about having kids next year. We will probably get an anonymous sperm donor' (Priscilla, 39); 'I would want a surrogate, a woman that I know. We would use both our sperm, four kids in total, two from each of us' (Kevin, 29); 'I may adopt a child as well. I would want to adopt a child from social services' (Mathapelo, 19).

Adoption was complicated because of concerns about the child's self-identity. Several participants disclosed that if they adopted a child, they would want to do so while the child was very young to prevent the child from knowing about his or her own adoption. While several participants had families in which individuals had raised and cared for siblings' children, few felt that taking a sibling's child to raise as one's own was viable.

Choices as to who would carry the child in lesbian relationships, or biologically father the child, were largely based on heteronormative gender roles. Feminine lesbians were more likely to carry a child in utero, and masculine-presenting men in gay relationships were more likely to donate sperm. However, as for Kevin (29), in gay relationships both men were able to provide sperm, and even when a gay feminine man was considered the 'woman' in the relationship, they considered multiplying the effects of their sperm. In Sibusisiwe's (42) lesbian relationship, the child carrier was the 'feminine' partner. Parents of children of previous opposite-sex relationships acknowledged their current partners' reproductive aspirations and tried to please them.

Blessings of a difficult past

The four participants we interviewed who already had children were no longer involved with their children's other biological parent. All regarded the relationship as a mistake or of no current substance, even if they were still on good terms with the former partner. Three of the four participants did not live with their children, but they felt no regret that they had had children. All children were welcomed by the families involved and, in some cases, the children enabled participants to live openly and with greater acceptance by their family. David (42) said, 'My grandmother asked for great-grandchildren. I tried to fulfil that for her, and I did have a daughter, but I was uncomfortable being with a woman. We stayed together for a year, but it didn't work. My daughter knows I'm gay as well.' When we asked, 'What did your grandmother say when you told her you were gay?', David replied, '[She said] since I had a child, I could do whatever I wanted. My mother says the same. As long as I am happy, my mother does not care.'

Not all cases ended like this. Some participants spoke of friends who were forced into relationships, and six associated such coercion with the risk of suicide. Many participants described their early childhood as difficult because some relatives had not accepted them and tried to force heteronormative behaviours, for example using gender-specific toys and clothes, and required heteronormative behaviour. Coming out, self-acceptance, and risks of violence in the wider community continued to plague most participants. Many found solace, spiritual strength and romantic partnerships in a community of LGBTIQA Christians.

The adage 'It takes a village to raise a child' shifts in meaning here – the 'village' may be a church community where gay men and lesbians find inspiration to think about how they might have their own children. Rather than through kinship and blood ties, relationships among gay and lesbian Christians in South Africa are quintessential 'chosen' families in the making. Whether children were unplanned, the result of a coerced or early sexual encounter, or intentional, they were seen as blessings from God: 'A child is a blessing from God Jehovah. They are necessary. No matter how much stress you have if you stay with a child, almost all you have [stress] will go away easily from you' (Lesedi, 19).

Lesedi said a child can be a blessing, enriching your life and impacting on your outlook. Blessings can take many forms and meanings. They can be gifts from God to the recipient, signifying a relationship with God and potentially legitimised by God in the same way that the recipient's own birth was. When asked, 'Would you ever change something about yourself,' most participants answered in the negative, elaborating that they were God's creations and did not need to be changed. This ensured or affirmed that their sexual orientation was morally legitimate to themselves and society. Priscilla (39) explained: 'God loves the fact that I am living the life God intended me to have.' Although LGBTIQA community members are often criticised as living wrongly or as a mistake, Priscilla was clear that God does not make mistakes. Lesedi (19) similarly concluded, 'He [God] loves me the way I am. He created me.'

In South Africa, a family without a child is often seen as incomplete, and childlessness may be considered a sign of something gone wrong. For Mpumalanga LGBTIQA Christians navigating sexual identity, religious identity and life in the wider community, a child is a marker of a complete family in line with society's and God's goals. Childlessness is a mark of difference between LGBTIQA peoples and heterosexuals, and for the latter, may signify why the former should be treated differently. Members of Ark of Joy aspire to have children by combining assistive reproductive technologies, social services and prior – sometimes difficult – childbearing experiences. Their prospective parental identities combine sexual and religious identities, sometimes through heteronormative gender roles. For these Christians, having a child of one's own, not necessarily biological, and being a child of God were both beautiful blessings in a world that historically has deemed everything to be wrong about them. Christianity, in this case, offered communal and idiomatic chances to show love and care.

Families, as illustrated above, are important social units. People turn to families for care and for emotional and financial support, and family members – especially parents – provide support for their children and grandchildren, based on values about their roles as parents and caregivers. Creating families allows for a sense of belonging and brings together the past, the present and the future, making connections with ancestral ties.

Making families is as critical in contexts of economic hardship, job precariousness and migration as it is in situations of relative comfort. The cases in this chapter illustrate the many ways by which people create families and attempt to sustain bonds of relatedness. Co-residence is one way of creating families and obligations. Having a child is one way of ensuring connections that are enduring, whether with the child or with the child and the father (and his family). However not all men want to support a child or keep in touch with the mother and/or child (Richter et al. 2010; see also Richter & Morrell 2006). The variables that affect whether the paternal family is involved include the age of the mother and father – the younger they are the more likely paternal kin will be involved, influencing reporting the pregnancy to the paternal family and the father's desire to be involved in raising the child. Marriage is a distant hope for most people, as discussions related to the payment of *lobola* illustrate (Posel et al. 2011).

Families are not defined by geographical location; they are about relationships and relatedness. While families and households are intertwined, families spill beyond the boundaries of households. Households in South Africa are often created pragmatically, influenced by structural factors that include migration, high levels of unemployment, poverty, and HIV and AIDS. Decisions made about livelihood influence both households and family creation.

Family is a critical support structure for most people, even when they live in separate households. We have illustrated that for women of limited means, especially without a partner, family support during pregnancy makes a difference to birthing decisions and experience. We have emphasised in this chapter the particular vulnerability of teenaged girls, women over 35, and migrant women to obstetric violence. Being a parent, for many, is a valued social identity, often redressing vulnerability associated with other identities – as a migrant, for instance, or as HIV positive, or as LGBTIQA. Raising a child may be hard work, but raising a child is also a way of 'growing', of caring for the self.

Note
1   Yeatman L, Did she abandon her baby? *Mail & Guardian*, 15 September 2017. Accessed 18 October 2019, https://mg.co.za/article/2017-09-15-00-did-she-abandon-her-baby

3 Family-keeping

Nolwazi Mkhwanazi and Lenore Manderson

Families are spaces where individuals come together to care for others and to receive care. Families, like households, are changing, as has already been noted. Family composition and membership change for various reasons: family members can be disowned if they act contrary to the values of the family; divorces and separations may sever family ties; marriages and births can create new families. Ultimately, families give individuals a sense of belonging through a shared lineage, a shared past or shared values, or at least an understanding of what those values are, even if they are not shared by all family members. And, as we have already suggested, family members play a major role in helping shape new families.

Care is central to ideas of family and is a central theme that runs through all the chapters of this book. What care means and how it manifests are not always apparent, nor is care necessarily experienced as positive. Obvious forms of care include day-to-day tasks to ensure that people are fed, washed and clothed, but other forms of care are less visible and often overlooked. This is particularly so when care is intergenerational. In asking how members of the family care for each other physically, emotionally and financially, we also need to attend to how care is enacted between generations. In this chapter, we explore how women and their partners, when present, make decisions about families and care. We describe support around adopting children, feeding infants, and sustaining family life. We also explore emerging patterns of self-care.

In Chapter 2, we discussed families in relation to physical, emotional and financial support, and discussed clinics and hospitals as forms of state-supported, institutionalised care. The case studies in this chapter focus on the care that happens between generations, especially between older women and their daughters who have become mothers themselves. This care attends not just to the immediate wellbeing of a child, but also to the wellbeing of generations on an affective level. But while intergenerational relationships are a critical source of support, especially in childcare, they are also often a source of tension (Moore 2013).

Grandmotherhood, motherhood and daughterhood are social identities of relatedness and are relational. Being a grandmother implies having been a mother; a mother is one who has had a child. However, these identities derive not simply from biological relatedness and chronology; they are awarded through acts of care. Identities enfold and inform one another (Blake 2017). Since they are awarded, they can be taken away when a person no longer fulfils the appropriate duties and responsibilities, or when someone chooses to withdraw from that identity. Identities are constantly negotiated between the self and others.

Every society has dominant ideas about parenthood and gender roles to which the majority adhere. These ideas differ according to culture, socioeconomic circumstances, geography, gender and generation. The ideas are also likely to change over time in response to local social, economic and political changes and global trends. Worldwide, generations often differ in their ideas regarding the behaviour that should accompany different life stages. These differences can lead to conflict, with generations pitted against each other, as was the case in South African townships in the late 1970s and 1980s, when young people inverted the social order of power and authority that had until then been in the hands of elders (Chikane 1986). Generational differences may also occur gradually, as Elena Moore (2013) describes for three generations of women in Cape Town, when ideas about motherhood, mothering, and maternal identity changed in response to socioeconomic and political circumstances. For the first generation, living under apartheid in the 1960s and 1970s, motherhood involved providing care for one's children, even if it meant leaving them for long periods of time to undertake paid work so that they had a secure home. For the second generation, mothering was not about marriage but about being a sole provider, and supporting family members to secure their better futures through education. For the third generation, mothering was an identity to be shared with a partner, thus enabling a mother to also pursue a career or life goals.

Young people who have just entered, or are soon to enter, parenthood have much to say about parenting. In their book *Books and Babies: Pregnancy and Young Parents in Schools*, based on their study in urban secondary schools in Durban and Cape Town in 2006 and 2007, Robert Morrell, Deevia Bhana and Tamara Shefer (2012) described the experiences of young mothers who returned to school after giving birth. In so doing, they reflected on existing policy and laws intended to safeguard a young mother's rights to education, and drew attention to dominant ideas among learners about parenthood. These ideas were largely congruent with the ideas of their parents. The majority believed that babies had no place in schools, that raising children was women's work, and that men should provide the resources to enable women to do so. Learners also strongly supported the idea that fathers be involved in a 'loving relationship' with their child. Contrary to teachers' views, many learners also supported young mothers being allowed to return to school to complete their education.

It seems contradictory that learners advocated that young mothers should be able to return to school, yet did not approve of the presence of babies at schools (that is, in a childcare centre on the premises). This contradiction reflects a dominant norm in South Africa of mothering and education as distinct spheres of life. Such an idea is captured in the document *Measures for the Prevention and Management of Learner*

Pregnancy, issued by the South African Department of Education (DoE 2007), which stated that pregnant learners may be 'required' to take leave of absence to have the child. No amount of time was specified, but the document stated that 'it is the view of the Department of Education that learners, as parents, should exercise full responsibility for parenting and that a period of absence of up to two years may be necessary for this purpose.' The document added: 'No learner should be re-admitted in the same year that they left the school due to pregnancy' (DoE 2007: 5). Thus this policy statement made clear two things: mothering should be confined to the home; and young women who returned to school immediately after giving birth, like Thandi (in Chapter 2), were 'irresponsible'.

Motherhood as a social identity is closely associated with the ways a woman cares for her child and the way she relates to others, but it is also an identity understood in the context of wider social relations. In 2011, the South African DoH adopted an exclusive six-month breastfeeding policy for all mothers, and emphasised that this was preferable to mixed feeding (often combining breastmilk and a thin porridge) (Nieuwoudt & Manderson 2018). However, many women in South Africa, for various reasons, cannot exclusively breastfeed for six months. In some contexts, mixed feeding may be expected of a 'good' mother by her family and the community to ensure that her child gets adequate nutrition. Sara Jewett Nieuwoudt undertook research with women in Soweto, with the aim of understanding their feeding decisions and practices (see Jewett Nieuwoudt 2019). In the following case study (3.1), drawing on in-depth interviews with the mothers of infants from 2016 to 2017, she illustrates how a woman's desire to be seen as a 'good' mother influences the infant-feeding decisions that she makes. Understanding the influence of ideologies and practices of mothering sheds light on the tensions that arise when 'good mother' feeding practices contradict those advised by health workers. Jewett Nieuwoudt illustrates the complexity and social implications of linking infant-feeding practices to ideal notions of motherhood, especially in a context where HIV stigma also affects decisions about infant feeding.

Case study 3.1

Being a good mother

Sara Jewett Nieuwoudt

Soweto starts for me with a turn at Exit 67 off the N1 South onto the Old Potch Road (now Chris Hani Road), and then a right towards Chris Hani Baragwanath Hospital, better known as 'Bara', where 20 000 infants are born every year. The behemoth was constructed in 1942. Soweto developed around it, accommodating swelling numbers of dispossessed people and migrants. Yet a white doctor could enter the academic tertiary hospital at the end of a journey from the leafy northern suburbs without ever driving down a township road or knowing the circumstances of how their patients – all African – were living during apartheid (1948–1994).

Little has changed. To get to the three-storey brick building where I work, I pass through a security entrance and a second boom gate. It was only when conducting field research that I drove down Soweto streets and entered the homes and lives of the women living there. These women included the three women I introduce below, all grappling with feeding their babies and being 'good' mothers in a community where 30 per cent of pregnant women test positive for HIV.

'I just try to be a good mother'

Molebogeng, my research assistant, and I first met Martha, aged 25 years, in the postnatal ward of a bustling community health clinic. She was eligible to participate in the study on infant-feeding influences – she was over 18 years old, she knew her HIV status, her infant was under six months, and she lived in Soweto – so we invited her to do so. We did not know that Martha had learned that she and her daughter, Karabo, had seroconverted two months after Karabo's birth, despite testing HIV negative twice during antenatal visits. Karabo was four months old when Martha first answered an interview questionnaire with us about infant feeding. At the time she was exclusively breastfeeding Karabo eight times a day. Karabo was six months old when Martha was interviewed for a second time. Martha explained that she just tried 'to be a good mother; I take care of her and I feed her well.' However, she was no longer breastfeeding:

> I feel good, but the problem is that I do not breastfeed her. I cannot mix-feed. When I used to express, I could only produce very little milk. I so badly wanted to breastfeed her, but I inevitably had to settle for formula. I am happy with having to give her formula, but the problem is that I really wanted to breastfeed her.

The desire to breastfeed that Martha showed has been highlighted by several researchers in relation to social ideals of good mothering, reinforced by a biomedical narrative that extols the intrinsic value of breastmilk (Mahon-Daly & Andrews 2002; Marshall et al. 2007). Martha's inability to produce milk was a way for her to legitimate not breastfeeding. She related her loss of milk to her distress on learning of Karabo's HIV status: 'I was very stressed out beyond words, and hence I couldn't even produce any breastmilk.' Martha's inability to breastfeed and its links to HIV, in this case emotionally, was interwoven with her story of trying to be a good mother. Her decision to shift to exclusive formula feeding at six months was in her mind the best alternative to breastmilk.

Martha's distress at being HIV positive was closely related to her experience of disclosure. When she told her boyfriend about her status and their daughter's status, he got very emotional, but, she explained, 'he honestly is ignorant about this HIV issue. He also doesn't want to get tested. He doesn't want to have anything to do with the HIV.' Beyond providing her with money to buy infant formula, he distanced himself from them. Martha told his sister, but neither she nor others in his family were supportive. Her disclosure to her own mother and sister was better, and they assist her as much as they can to raise Karabo. Martha leaves Karabo with her sister when she goes to school, part time.

Understandings of what constituted 'good feeding' changed how Martha understood good mothering of her infant daughter. For many mothers, including Martha, mixed feeding was a key issue. Martha emphasised 'I cannot mix-feed' in relation to feeding Karabo 'well'. However, she had not always thought this. In her interview at four months, Martha explained that when she gave birth she started breastfeeding immediately, as do most women in South Africa (Du Plessis et al. 2016). However, when she went home, she succumbed to her mother's pressure to mix-feed and started adding porridge to Karabo's diet at one month old; by four months she had given her daughter gripe water, rooibos tea and semi-solid foods as well as breastmilk. Martha highlighted the importance of being a good daughter and adhering to family norms: 'My mother tried to encourage me to feed her solids so that Karabo could pick up weight, but I decided to stick with the dietician's plan.' Her mother persisted, and Martha finally did 'succumb' and gave her daughter solid foods until she (the infant) was admitted to the hospital with chronic diarrhoea.

Martha began to rely on the hospital dietician's advice when Karabo was diagnosed with HIV. Her mother, too, came to trust the dietician's advice about exclusive feeding, including that breastmilk was sufficient and the 'baby's tummy was still too tiny for solid food.' The rapid shifts in Martha's infant-feeding beliefs and practices during the first six months, in the context of coming to terms with her HIV status, left me feeling that she was still uncertain, relying on outsiders to confirm she was as 'good' a mother as she was trying to be. When we asked how she fed Karabo compared with other babies in her family, she explained that Karabo was 'tiny and perhaps I am not feeding her well, but they [the nurses] have stated that she is picking up weight.' Now that Karabo was six months old, Martha was about to enter the next phase of complementary feeding, with its own set of challenges.

The concept that a baby's growth is a reflection of a mother's ability was strongly embedded in interviews with mothers, healthcare workers and family members. Naledi, another HIV-positive mother, also saw her infant's growth as a reflection of her feeding decisions: 'I feel happy, his body is developing well and it shows that he is growing.' Naledi had exclusively breastfed her son, Tonderai, for six months. An immigrant from Zimbabwe, she was currently living with her boyfriend, their older child and Tonderai. Like Martha, Naledi had to actively resist pressures to mix-feed as the norm, both in the family and the local Zimbabwean community. However, she took courage from the way Tonderai was developing to demonstrate that she was a good mother – this was evidence that her feeding choices were right. For her, the clinic advice about milk sufficiency was critical: 'I was happy with the decision. I felt that it was the right decision to make and if I didn't know any better, I would have thought that my baby would starve from the breastmilk alone, I would have thought the breastmilk alone would never be enough.'

Family and community concepts of womanhood influenced women's infant-feeding practices. Though Naledi's boyfriend supported her with Tonderai, her immediate family members had called her lazy not to mix-feed her first infant. She accepted this label with humour as a way of coping: 'I am very lazy to cook and my family would also ask me why I wasn't making food for the baby. I was very lazy.' Accepting this derogatory label was part of her strategy to breastfeed her firstborn child, which she did for 18 months. Exclusively breastfeeding Tonderai was easier, as she knew her HIV status before becoming pregnant, as did her boyfriend, and he supported her decision to breastfeed for up to one year. He also supported giving their baby Nevirapine syrup to reduce the risk of transmission. With this support, it was easier for her to deflect questions from neighbours. She explained that babies in the community are typically introduced to solids in the first month:

> At about two–three weeks they'd start making porridge for them, but sometimes you look at the baby and you can see that they are not healthy and they'd ask me whether or not I have started feeding porridge to my baby and I'd tell them no, my baby is fine. They'd also say that my baby looks like I am feeding him solid food already, and I would add that my baby is fine.

When neighbours challenged her, Naledi persisted: 'I would say that my baby gets his fill from my breastmilk alone and all I have to do is to make sure that I have a balanced diet such that I can produce enough milk to his satisfaction.'

Other mothers did not have supportive partners or an easy time dealing with accusations of being lazy. Busi, a healthcare worker, described how her husband accused her of being too lazy to cook as the reason for refusing to mix-feed her children. She explained, 'I was not lazy. It was [too] early for them to eat food and I was at home because my maternity leave was four months. So [my milk] was enough'. Despite her protestations, her husband bullied her into mixed feeding all three of their children at five months, when she had to return to work. In addition to accusing her of being lazy, he drew on his own experience of helping to raise his siblings when his mother was working. He had been responsible for feeding his younger brothers and sisters, and he believed their own children should be raised the same way. Gill Seidel (2004) has noted how descriptions of 'lazy' mothers have extended into South Africa's healthcare setting.

As Martha and Naledi explain, the idea of good feeding originates from family traditions and community norms, which are policed by gender expectations of what it means to be a good mother. Busi's husband actively denigrated the knowledge she brought from the clinic. Particularly when her children were crying, he would say, 'He is hungry. Hey, you are coming with this stuff for the clinic every time – clinic says this, clinic says that.' He accused her of privileging clinic advice over the hunger of her own child. While she was unable to completely follow clinic advice, Busi described her attempts to circumvent her husband to apply her understandings of best feeding practices. She left her children with another woman when she returned to work, until, at the age of three, they were able to go to crèche, and during this time, she provided expressed breastmilk: 'Ja, it was very nice because the husband didn't see what's what. See what was happening. I expressed and the old lady just gave porridge. That food and then it was milk.'

Women often described cooperative caregiving for working mothers, whereby infants were left with family members, neighbours or at a crèche. Depending on the relationship they had with caregivers, this could become a way to sustain desired feeding decisions, such as Busi continuing to give her children breastmilk or Martha's sister helping to give her daughter formula and medication while Martha was studying. Placing infants in the care of others has been seen as a reason some HIV-positive mothers opt for formula, because they do not trust that the caregiver will abide by their decisions (Zulliger et al. 2013). However, the cases here point to positive features of women helping women, away from the male gaze, particularly in Busi's case. A common feature of cooperative caregiving was that it was a realm dominated by female relationships.

Unlike Martha and Naledi, Busi did not have to navigate decisions about the HIV risks of breastfeeding. However, she observed the challenges of making infant-feeding choices in a community that was hypersensitive about HIV, even for HIV-negative women:

> Most of the people visit, they want to see whether they are HIV positive or not. Because they know, those who are not breastfeeding are HIV positive. They don't know every mother can breastfeed, HIV positive or HIV negative. You can breastfeed. And they don't know that ... Ja those people like to talk about HIV with the community. She wants to sit alone in the house and tell stories.

The fear of being stigmatised by the community was not just about infant feeding (mixed or exclusive), but also about what this choice signified. As Busi explained, exclusive feeding, particularly using formula, was understood within the community as unique to people with HIV. The idea that HIV-positive women can breastfeed is not understood fully in this community, it would seem.

In South Africa, the ideal of exclusive breastfeeding for six months has problems. Early in my research, I interviewed a prominent paediatrician who had worked in the field of child malnutrition for over 20 years, many of them at Bara. He reflected on the advice many pregnant woman receive in public-health settings: 'The message has always been about breastfeeding is best, and for me that's as a hollow as saying eating food is good for you. It's exactly the equivalent, because what does "breastfeeding is best" mean?' The idea of 'best' was taken up by women like Busi, Naledi and Martha as a marker of the kind of mothers they would like to be. Naledi succeeded; Martha did her best, until she was no longer able; and Busi also did her best, but was unable to fully avert social pressures once she returned to work.

All three women associated infant feeding with their value as mothers. While some scholars have argued that the public-health narrative of 'breast is best' has made breastfeeding a moral imperative (Marshall et al. 2007), all three women highlighted the fact that 'best feeding practice' is highly contested. In Soweto, mixed feeding of any kind – breastmilk and formula and solids – remains a strong norm. The advice women receive from antenatal clinics to feed exclusively is not widely accepted, and exclusive feeding was associated with HIV. Depending on how mothers felt about HIV, whether they had disclosed (if positive), and the support they received from immediate family, strongly influenced their ability to maintain exclusive feeding, as Tanya Doherty et al. (2006) also found. Fears of actual HIV transmission, the fear of being identified as HIV positive (fear of stigma), and mixed-feeding norms acted as barriers to exclusive feeding then and continue to do so over a decade later.

While all three women exerted agency, women like Busi were not able to fully enact their desired feeding decisions. Martha's initial decision to mix-feed illustrates how family influenced her concept of what was good. The lengths to which family members went to change mother's decisions, invoking history, tradition and gender roles, point to the social meanings of infant feeding, well beyond meeting the nutritional needs of an infant (see Marshall et al. 2007). Soweto – as Martha, Naledi and Busi describe it – remains a place where HIV is a cause for gossip and exclusion. Infant-feeding choices are interpreted as signifiers of one's status; they become an involuntary disclosure to the community. Unless practices like exclusive breastfeeding are normalised for all women, a certain degree of individual resilience and family support, as experienced by Naledi, will be needed for mothers in Soweto to meet the standards of what public health defines as a 'good mother'.

How mothers feed their infants is not simply about making sure they grow and meet the desired measurements for their percentile. Infant feeding is a form of communication between mother and baby, and from the mother to the people around her. Infant feeding is also an act of creating a person, a way of sustaining life and family-keeping. While the state's aim in promoting exclusive breastfeeding to reduce infant mortality is also about sustaining life, women's understanding and the state's understanding of how best to sustain life are very different. This is reflected in the practices that each advocate: mixed feeding and exclusive feeding respectively.

While medically, exclusive breastfeeding may be ideal, infant feeding largely depends on the material circumstances of the mother. The women described above live in poverty. As is the case for many African women today and for generations before them, returning to income-generating activities after giving birth in order to contribute to household resources may be paramount. To do so they must leave their child in the care of someone else. Consequently, the decision to mix-feed is a pragmatic one.

Infant-feeding practices are shaped by different life experiences and biographies. For many women, especially of older generations, for whom hunger was not uncommon, solid food satiates, and breastmilk alone is not seen to be sufficient to sustain infants. For a child to grow and thrive, many believe, a mother needs to boost the child's health with medicines, feed the child solid foods, and provide liquids to quench thirst. In many contexts of poverty, big babies are perceived as healthy and happy (Scheper-Hughes 1992; Majombozi 2015).

The control and distribution of knowledge and practices regarding reproduction are contested in every society. Women don't just accept that knowledge passively. They actively engage in decisions about their bodies and about their children. In response to conflicting information given by public health officials on the one hand, and individuals in their lives – especially grandmothers – on the other, mothers weigh the two and draw on their own experiences to decide how to act. Despite the constraints under which women may live, they exercise some agency in shaping their reproductive lives. In the next case study (3.2), Nirvana Pillay draws on her ethnographic research on adolescent pregnancy and agency in the township of Alexandra in Johannesburg (see Pillay 2019). This case study specifically focuses on three young women to examine how their families responded to an unanticipated pregnancy, and how the young mothers and babies were cared for and absorbed within existing, extended and new family networks. The three mothers – Nobuhle (aged 18 years), Ayanda (aged 19 years) and Betty (aged 20 years) – were interviewed three times each between September 2016 and August 2017, and Pillay also interviewed a significant other person in their life: mother, grandmother or father of the baby. The case study illustrates how young women exercise agency in decisions about how and by whom their children are raised. It shows how three women from quite different family constellations and circumstances adjust, shift and reorient their young families in response to structural constraints and the constantly changing demands of everyday living.

Case study 3.2

'I don't want friends … I have family'

Nirvana Pillay

For young mothers who have no support from state and other social, educational and development agencies following an unplanned or mistimed pregnancy, families play a crucial role in their lives.

Writing of multiple generations and family members can be confusing. So, to clarify: below, I use the term 'young mother' to refer to the protagonist of the story – Nobuhle, Ayanda or Betty; I refer to her mother as 'mother', her mother's mother as 'grandmother', and her baby as 'son/daughter'.

Nobuhle's story

Nobuhle was 18 years old when I first met her at the Health Centre. She was with her 6-week old daughter Titzi. Nobuhle was 17 when she conceived, 18 when she gave birth. She passed matric at the end of 2015 at the age of 17 with a diploma, and became pregnant soon after writing her examination. Passing her final year of secondary study with a diploma means that Nobuhle is not eligible for tertiary studies in South African universities; she would have to upgrade her matriculation to study further. Nobuhle aspires to do this, and to pursue a social work degree. When we first met, Nobuhle was in a long-term relationship with Solly, Titzi's father. They had been together for two years when Nobuhle conceived.

When I first met Nobuhle, I was struck by her confidence, energy, ease and pride in her new infant. Describing her health during her pregnancy, Nobuhle animatedly stated, 'I was able to run very fast and I would jump off things, I was very active, I was very hyper, my mom was always scared, I would climb on top of the bed … jump.' In the first interview she seemed determined to overcome the challenges presented to her as a young mother. But as we got to know each other, Nobuhle was not always this positive and excited. As our relationship deepened I began to make sense of her life, her relationships, struggles and dreams. In our time of contact, Nobuhle began with the faith that her relationship with Titzi's father would endure, and that they would raise Titzi together and begin a little family of their own. She was certain that Solly and his family would pay *inhlawulo* to her family, and perform the traditional rite of acknowledging paternity and accepting the new baby into the family. She was sympathetic to Solly's not yet having paid *inhlawulo* because he and his family had insufficient money; both Mavis, her mother, and Nobuhle allowed him to visit Titzi even though the damages were not paid. However, Nobuhle grew increasingly wary of the future, after being physically abused by Solly a number of times.

Nobuhle and Titzi lived with her mother, Mavis (41), in a single rented room in Alexandra. Her nuclear family includes Mavis, her father (separated from Mavis since 2008), who also lives in Alexandra, and an older brother (22) at school and living in Limpopo with Mavis's family. Nobuhle, Titzi and Mavis live on a household income of approximately R3 000, which Mavis earns, and the Child Support Grant. Nobuhle gets occasional work at a clothing store, too, after losing a part-time job at a fashion store because of absenteeism due to one of Solly's beatings. Solly offers occasional but irregular support in the form of food or clothes for Titzi. Nobuhle's father also occasionally gives his ex-wife and daughter money for food or meat, but again this is not reliable.

During the year, Nobuhle told me of her battles and victories as a young mother, her ongoing struggle to find employment, and the enduring love and support she has received from her mother. In this time, Nobuhle had to negotiate the end of school with disappointing results; a pregnancy and birth; a traumatic and stressful love relationship; having and losing a job; and the endless pursuit of finding employment in an economy unkind to young people in general, and particularly challenging for young mothers. Other family members and Solly step in and step out; nothing sustains their commitment to the household. Hence it is the mother–daughter dyad and the strength of their bond that adapts and meets the changing context of their lives, including the joint planning and decision-making around Titzi's wellbeing and care.

Ayanda's story

When we met, Ayanda was 19 years old, and her daughter, Lumile, was 1 year old. Ayanda was 17 when she conceived, 18 when she gave birth. She had completed matriculation at the end of 2014 at the age of 17 and found out that she was pregnant soon after. Ayanda had an incomplete matriculation result as she did not write the examination for two subjects, and spent part of 2015 upgrading her results so that she could pursue tertiary studies. Lumile's father, Nde, is 22, and he and Ayanda had been together for 4 years when Ayanda became pregnant. Although Nde wanted Ayanda to keep the baby, he chose to leave their relationship. He has no contact with either Ayanda or his daughter Lumile.

Ayanda was fiery, easily able to articulate her views and confident with me from our first meeting. She exuded ambition and drive, and did not seem deterred by life's difficulties. At no point in our conversations did she describe sadness, despair or disappointment, despite the many challenges and difficulties she has experienced. Her mother had died in 2002 from breast cancer and her father died in 2008. She was her parents' only child, but she refers to her cousins with whom she now lives with her grandmother, Faith (62), as her younger brothers.

Ayanda has lived with Faith since 2010, along with her aunt (mother's sister) and her aunt's sons (14 and 12 years old), in a one-room dwelling in Alexandra owned by Faith. Ayanda and Faith have a close relationship, with Faith investing in Ayanda through expensive private education and providing her with unconditional support despite her disappointment in the pregnancy. The household income consists of approximately R7 000 earned by Faith, and ad hoc money provided from Ayanda's aunt's income as an occasional domestic worker. Ayanda receives the Child Support Grant. Their monthly income is above average for a household in Alexandra, but it is still a constant struggle to meet household needs, including for baby Lumile. When we met a second time in January 2017, Ayanda told me that Faith had just retired and that Lumile was no longer living with her in Alexandra, but was with her second aunt and her husband in Rustenberg. Her aunt had no children of her own, and was happy to support Ayanda to allow her to continue her studies and look for work, all of which were difficult to manage while caring for a baby. Ayanda had enrolled at a local college to study human resource management and was working for a commission-based sales company. She had great hopes that with drive, commitment and hard work she could earn good commissions and eventually lead her own team.

It is not uncommon for babies and children in South African urban townships to be raised by family members outside the township, as Lumile was. Childcare is often onerous and stressful for mothers in poor urban areas; crèches and family support are limited; and lack of resources often drive the decision to bring in support from the wider family network in caregiving (see also Mkhwanazi's case study 2.1). What was striking about Ayanda's case, however, was the fluid way in which Lumile and Ayanda are held within the wider family network, Ayanda's pragmatic approach to Lumile's care by an aunt, and how the entire family seeks to support Ayanda as a potential breadwinner. Ayanda's own determination, and her pragmatic approach to Lumile's care, set her apart from the dominant narrative of the passive teenaged mother (see Mkhwanazi 2017). Lumile was absorbed into a second family in Rustenberg, while maintaining her family in Alexandra, and her connection to them. Ayanda is confident that Lumile knows of their mother–daughter bond, even though she calls Ayanda's aunt 'Mamma':

> Ai, that one, she'll never forget me, there is no way. Because when they came she could see I know this person, she was busy staring at me and then the next thing she wanted me to carry her and then from there I couldn't go out without going with her … if I go to the shop, I must take her with me and she didn't sleep if I'm not sleeping at night. We have to switch off the lights and she makes sure that I'm right next to her you see, ah she won't forget me that one.

Betty's story

Betty was 20 years old and her son Mpho 6 months old when we first met. Betty was 18 when she conceived, 19 when she gave birth. She was in Grade 11 when she found out about her pregnancy and decided to drop out of school during her matriculation year, in the month Mpho was born. Mpho's father, Junior (27), and Betty have a complicated relationship. Their relationship started in the Eastern Cape where they met at school; they parted ways for a while, and then reconnected when they both ended up in Alexandra. They had been together for five years when Betty became pregnant. Junior had encouraged Betty to keep the baby, but Betty was uncertain of their relationship status and constantly worried about his infidelity. Junior was clear that they now only had a shared relationship with Mpho, and when we last met, Betty, too, was clear that their relationship as a couple was over.

Unlike Nobuhle and Ayanda, Betty was withdrawn and quiet, and very sad the first few times we met. She struggled with her relationship with Junior. The strain of having a baby without her own income weighed heavily on her, and she had difficulty finding employment so she could have financial independence.

Betty and Mpho live with her uncle (mother's brother) and aunt (mother's sister, although Betty spoke of her as her sister in our conversations), the aunt's two children, and her grandmother in a house owned by her grandmother. There were therefore seven members of the household. Betty described her living arrangements as adaptable and temporary. She lived with her mother while she was pregnant and shortly after giving birth, while she was cared for, and there learnt the basics of infant care (bathing, feeding) from her mother. She then moved in with her aunt and uncle so that she and Mpho could have more room. Unlike the earlier cases, where the families were split between 'homes' (Limpopo and Eastern Cape), almost all of Betty's family resided in Alexandra. The family households are supported primarily by Betty's aunt, who works full time, and Betty's mum, who works part time as a domestic worker. Betty did not know how much either earned. By the end of my fieldwork, Betty had found a job in the deli counter of a local supermarket. She was a very different young woman at our last meeting – happy, chatty, and confident. She was clear that her relationship with Junior was over, but she was pleased that he was still involved in Mpho's life and she was keen to encourage and nurture this.

For Betty, financial independence was the major source of distress in early motherhood, and not the unplanned baby Mpho or her difficult relationship with Junior. When Betty started her new job, she left Mpho with a caregiver to whom she pays R450 a month. When she came home late from work, or needed to leave early to work, a family member would step in and fetch Mpho from the caregiver and bath and feed him.

Betty's story illustrates the support networks intrinsic to large extended families. Her use of the terms 'brother' and 'sister', not 'uncle' and 'aunt', reflects the fluidity of nuclear families, shaped by roles and not by genealogy, and constituted in multiple, flexible ways. Mpho was absorbed into a wide family network, where his mother's mother and her siblings rallied round and supported Betty, particularly when she was financially dependent on them. Junior's support became peripheral to the maintenance of the family and household. Yet Betty actively encouraged Junior's relationship with his son, and acknowledged that his support, although ad hoc and inconsistent, was valued: 'When he asks me to bring the baby I don't have a problem, I bring the baby to him. When he wants to come and see the baby I don't have a problem, he come and see the baby.'

Nobuhle's, Ayanda's and Betty's stories tell a larger story about the families and households of young mothers and their babies in a poor urban township. Each story shows how love, care and generosity are provided to young mothers and their children within uncertain and fragile household economies. Studies in South Africa have documented how families, households and their networks come together to offer care in times of stress. This happened even when unanticipated events strain existing scarce resources, for example when an unplanned and mistimed pregnancy potentially limits the young mother's chance of education and getting employed (see Mkhwanazi & Bhana 2017). Parents and caregivers dream that their children will help their families out of hardship and poverty, and, even in constrained circumstances, families work to accommodate unanticipated events.

The fathers of Nobuhle's and Betty's babies also represent alternative narratives to those of absent young fathers. Although their relationships with the young mothers did not endure, in both cases the men remained committed to their babies, and offered some support in the form of Pampers (disposable nappies), food and occasional cash, as well as regular visits to see them. While both families would have liked the men to observe *inhlawulo*, they were willing to be flexible to sustain the father–baby relationship (see also Nkani 2017). Further, while men in general, and fathers in particular, are present in these stories, the dynamics of care and support are strongly gendered, with older women offering the bulk of financial and caregiving support for their daughters, granddaughters and infants.

In the preceding chapter, we saw that the birth of a child is often accompanied by decisions about who will care for the child and how the child will be cared for. These decisions may or may not be negotiated outright, but the people who converge to help care for the child become family. Over the last three decades, the majority of families created after the birth of a child to a teenaged mother are often matrifocal. Thus research on teenaged parenting has mainly focused on teenage mothers and their families. Even so, there has been increasing interest in the fathers of children of teenaged mothers, and their involvement in young families (Bhana & Nkani 2014;

Chili & Maharaj 2015; Enderstein & Boonzaier 2013; Swartz & Bhana 2009). Previous studies omitted the genitor's involvement because most genitors denied paternity or they were unable to pay damages and so were denied access to the child. Mark Hunter (2005) suggests that men commonly denied paternity not because they did not want to be involved in the lives of their children, but owing to high rates of unemployment, they were financially unable to 'meet the accepted social role of fatherhood' as a provider. Recent researchers have shown that although genitors are still unable to pay *inhlawulo*, young fathers especially want to be involved in the lives of their children (Mvune et al. 2019). In addition, teenaged mother's families often accommodate the father's and his kin's desire to be involved in caring for the child (Mkhwanazi & Block 2016; Nkani 2017). This is apparent in a number of case studies in this book, and suggests that practices of relatedness, belonging and care are changing.

For many pregnant African women, neither termination nor adoption is considered an option. As described for Ayanda and Lumile in case study 3.1, child circulation in African families where other family members raise children is relatively common, whether or not children's biological parents are alive. Formal adoption, however, may be viewed with mistrust and scepticism, primarily associated with concerns of ancestral and family belonging. The number of formal adoptions taking place in African communities is low. Indeed, some provincial departments of social development have been reported to be constructively preventing the adoption of African children.

In the next case study (3.3), drawing on ethnographic research conducted in the Gauteng province in 2013 and 2014, Deirdre Blackie discusses perceptions of adoption in African communities. She focuses on two young men who found out later in life that they had been adopted after being abandoned by their birth mothers. As she demonstrates, beliefs about family, children and belonging affect where and with whom orphans and abandoned children are placed.

Case study 3.3

Connected

Deirdre Blackie

I met Xolani at a mall on the outskirts of Soweto. He had been referred to me by a child-protection organisation he had recently contacted to try to find out who his birth mother was. Xolani was 22, confident and friendly, and appeared to take great care of his appearance; I later learnt that he was a personal trainer and was looking for employment at a newly opened gym. As I started talking to him about my research on child abandonment, his confidence dissipated, the energy seemed to seep out of his body, and he slowly and silently started to cry. This was not the first time I had experienced this when talking to a young man about his adoption and recently discovered abandonment by his birth mother.

Child abandonment has increased rapidly in South African cities since the end of apartheid in 1994, with child-welfare organisations estimating that more than 3 000 children are abandoned each year.[1] Reasons cited include rapid urbanisation, poverty and high levels of gender abuse towards women (Blackie 2014), and restrictive legislation that has particular effects in the case of teenage pregnancy and for women who lack documentation of residence. Although a woman of any age can consent to an abortion, she must be 18 years or older to consent to her child's adoption, and she can access the South African child-protection system only as a citizen. The Registry of Adoptable Children and Adoptive Parents (RACAP) in November 2013 revealed that of the unmatched children listed, over 60 per cent were abandoned, and less than 40 per cent were formally consented for adoption by their biological parents or family. This majority of abandoned children in the child-protection system has remained consistent over the past five years. However, the number of adoptions has declined significantly. Only 1 349 adoptions took place in 2016, down from 2 840 in 2004, while foster-care numbers have soared to more than 500 000 children over the same period (NACSA 2017). High levels of abandonment and low levels of adoption, and conflicting views and perceptions on these practices, point to a need for a better understanding of the political and social context of this situation.

Abandoned and disconnected

Xolani was found on the streets of a suburb of Soweto, wrapped in newspaper to stay warm, not far from where he lives now with his adopted mother.

Abandonment appears to be increasing, each year and in the colder winter months. Reasons for this include a lack of support or social services for women not born in South Africa from the departments of Health, Justice, Home Affairs, Police and Social Development. Newspaper articles on child abandonment reveal that most abandonments occur just after birth or in a child's first year of life (Blackie 2014). Safe sites include baby safes,[2] hospitals and crèches, but state hospitals have improved their protocols and security, making safer abandonment extremely difficult for women who choose this option. The majority of children are abandoned at unsafe sites – toilets, sewers, rubbish sites, dustbins, landfills, parks, and the open veld. An estimated two of every three babies abandoned die (NACSA 2017), and those who survive are often premature, have some level of dehydration, hypothermia, infection, and animal and insect wounds due to the environment in which they were abandoned.

Xolani was taken to a hospital, and after three months he was adopted by a nurse who had cared for him over this time. She did not tell him he was adopted.

However, following her death, Xolani started to feel ostracised by the people he thought were his biological family, and he was told of his adoption:

> My mom loved me so much, but she couldn't tell me. She did what she thought was best for me. After she died, her sister started acting up on me. I asked her why is everything changing now, we used to spend weekends together, they would come around or I would go to them, but now they don't come anymore. That's when she told me, 'I have sad news for you, you are adopted.' I didn't know what to do, I didn't have anyone to speak to, I felt completely alone. My girlfriend helped me, I have a daughter with her who is nine months old, but I feel like I have nothing to live for. My daughter looks like me, she is my own flesh and blood, she has made me very happy. I don't know who my parents are. The abandonment, I am still dealing with that. I met with the people at the welfare and they told me there are many reasons that people do this. Perhaps they were not from this country, maybe she was very young, they told me a lot of things. They found me near Mapetla, it's just an area, I want to go there, maybe next week, it's all new to me, I'm still dealing with it. I am a very emotional person. I want to find out more. There is a possibility that I find out who I am, where I am from, my culture. I don't know who I am.

I spoke to a number of young people who had only discovered their adoption, and prior abandonment, on reaching adulthood, and all revealed a painful and ongoing embodied experience akin to extreme 'social suffering' (Farmer 1996; Scheper-Hughes 1992). When I asked Thabo, another young man from Soweto, where he feels the pain, he told me – tapping forcefully on his chest with his fingers – 'Everywhere, it's like being stabbed in the heart, over and over again.' These young people felt that they no longer belonged in the family into which they had been adopted, and expressed complicated emotions of alienation and rejection. Thabo explained:

> I was distraught. I was confused about who I was before, but finding out that I wasn't even who I thought I was [shaking his head]. These are not my people, I am not their child. It was so confusing, the thoughts in my head, it was really messy inside me. That day [he found out he was adopted] broke a crack, and things haven't been the same since.

Abandonment caused a huge sense of loss and rejection. Many young men spoke of not wanting to live; some had attempted suicide. They felt disconnected from their families and their ancestors. Xolani believed that he would not be able to perform his traditional duties of husband and father, linked to the paying of *lobola*. He wished to marry his girlfriend, pay damages for his daughter, and allow her to use his clan name. He believed his abandonment and lack of connection to his agnatic line prevented him from doing these things:

> I want to know if I am a Zulu, or a Tswana or Shangaan. I believe in ceremonies, I have to perform ceremonies for my baby, but to do that I have to find my dad. At the moment, we are using her mother's surname. I should go to her family and pay *ilobola*. If I had my father's name, I would use that name. I can be able to go and *ukuhlawala* [the act of paying *inhlawulo*], to pay damages for my child. I want my baby to use my real surname.

The cultural divide

Men had many concerns about their unknown ancestry and this had an impact on their wellbeing. Their concerns stemmed from the belief that ancestors would care for children only of the same blood line. Abandoned children would be cared for by community members but could not participate in family rituals as this would displease the family's ancestors:

> The community prefers it if abandoned children stay with them, but they cannot make them part of their family through adoption. The child will be looked after, given food, clothes, sent to school, but if they are doing any rituals as a family, the child must leave and go and sleep at someone else's house that night. If they stay, the ancestors will see them sleeping there and be angry, because they don't belong. Most people try and help young people to find their families, but there is a line that cannot be crossed. (social worker, Alexandra)

This sentiment was supported by the Commissioner for Traditional Leadership Disputes and Crimes in KwaZulu-Natal, who stated publicly, 'It would take years before there was a flexibility of mind about adoption among most South Africans. We would have to have a big indaba [meeting] before it could be accepted. Ancestral spirits look after their relatives and no-one else. In our religion, in our culture, this thing is ring-fenced.'[3]

This fear of family rejection often results in adoptive parents withholding knowledge of adoption status:

> This young black couple are wanting to adopt. Neither of their families know that they are wanting to do this. The couple believe that they are taking a risk with their ancestors, but they are desperate for a child. They plan to pretend that the child is theirs, and not to visit their family whilst they are supposedly pregnant. They have agreed that when he has grown up, they will do some kind of ritual to help him, but in the meantime, no one needs to know. (Rose)

Although 'informal adoption' is common, whereby children are assimilated into families following the death of a parent or abandonment, people resist a formal legal approach, primarily due to concerns of ancestral and family belonging. The resistance to formal adoption is evident throughout South Africa, but especially in KwaZulu-Natal. This province has the highest number of orphans countrywide, yet only eight adoptions took place in 2016. The primary child-protection strategies focus on family reunification/preservation and foster care: adoption is not even mentioned (*Daily Maverick* 23 August 2017). The constructive prevention of adoption was highlighted by non-governmental social workers and child-protection organisations throughout my fieldwork, and took the form of accusations of child trafficking to adoption social workers and adoptive parents, intimidating birth mothers and biological families who had formally consented to adoption. This is despite the fact that both the South African Children's Act (No. 38 of 2005) and The Hague Adoption Convention, to which South Africa is a signatory, state that children should grow up in a family environment and that permanency is preferable to temporary measures.

People commonly believe that taking a child of unrelated ancestry and introducing them legally into a new family could cause problems for both the child and the adoptive parents, as this is not a recognised form of kinship creation amongst their ancestors. Equally, formally relinquishing one's parental rights so that a child may be deemed adoptable is seen as problematic, leading many children to be abandoned into the formal child-protection system (Blackie 2014). State-employed social workers, police officers and nurses referred to the abandoning mothers as 'immoral' or 'criminal', and frequently mentioned concerns around their 'spiritual wellbeing'. They believed that a mother's choice to abort or abandon her child would result in extreme suffering at the hands of her ancestors. Midwives in Gauteng revealed that these concerns were not just for the mothers, but for anyone involved in abortion or adoption. If a person helped a woman abort, or was complicit in placing a child for adoption (for example, by phoning an adoption social worker on behalf of a birth mother), they would be 'guilty by association' and might also by punished by their ancestors. The challenge is that family reunification/preservation is not possible for a child who has been abandoned anonymously.

Healing the divide

Given cultural concerns around adoption, I interviewed a number of traditional healers or *tangoma* (plural of *sangoma*) as part of my fieldwork. More than half had children who had been abandoned with them by unrelated individuals, and who they were bringing up as their own. Most believed that the abandoning mother saw them as spiritual individuals who could assist their children to engage with their ancestors, despite their abandonment. Whilst all *tangoma* were critical, they understood why abandonment occurred and in some instances played the role of surrogate parent:

> My young girl was left with me when she was hardly a month old. The woman who abandoned her told me that she was going into town, but she never returned [this was in rural KwaZulu-Natal]. My mother and I informed our *induna* [an advisor or leader], who told us to take the child to the police. We went to the police station to do an affidavit and the police asked us if we were willing to keep the baby, so we took her home. The mother is not related to us at all, so when we got home, my mother and I took a chicken and *imphepo* [natural plant burnt as incense], and then we *ubigile*, we announced the baby to the ancestors. We asked the ancestors to accept this baby and to help us in raising her. We adopted this baby and gave her the surname Isikaya, our name. We got birth certificates and we brought her up as our own child. She is now doing matric, she is well behaved, better than my own children [he laughs], she appreciates being taken care of. (*Sangoma* Baba Ndaba)

The *tangoma* advised that if a child were found abandoned, the person who finds the child should consult their ancestors immediately to assist the child 'find their way' from a spiritual perspective. This was also considered necessary if a child was born out of wedlock. They explained that ancestors have a certain view on how and which children would be recognised as part of a family. For a child to be accepted, it would need to be introduced to its father's ancestors. Introduction to the ancestors of its mother's family, or of a different and unrelated family, would cause confusion and consternation amongst the ancestors. This is not to say that a child cannot be introduced to the ancestors, but that the ancestors must be consulted to assist the child to find his or her spiritual home:

> I did the right process, by announcing the baby to my ancestors, so there wasn't a problem. Unlike if I had taken this baby without announcing it, and just lived with it. To the ancestors, this would have been a problem. It is the same if girl children have babies in your home. Those children need to be announced to the ancestors, because babies that are recognised by the ancestors in this home are babies that are born by the daughter-in-law, not by the daughters of this house. Remember his father is from another surname and another clan. This is why you see so many of the girl child's children landing up in criminal behaviours and in jail, because they have not been announced to the ancestors. (*Sangoma* Baba Ndaba)

I was repeatedly told by community members that children could search for their ancestors all of their lives with no success. Some may engage the help of a diviner to tell them where to find their father's family, and they would then need to ask this family to intercede on their behalf with their ancestors. However, *tangoma* had a different view. They told me that ancestors are with you from the moment you are born, even if you do not know your father's name. The ancestors may not engage with you directly, because you don't know how to address them, but they are always with you. If a child is adopted into a new family and announced to that family's ancestors, both sets of ancestors can connect with each other, as the child's ancestors are already with him or her, and the family's ancestors have been called appropriately. No *sangoma* I spoke to opposed formal adoption, although they were concerned if the ancestors of the child and the adoptive parents were unrelated. They suggested that this could be particularly difficult for boys who needed their ancestors for important kinship rituals such as marriage and the acknowledgement of their own children. Consultation and allowing the ancestors to guide families through these difficult times, with the help and support of a *sangoma*, was seen as the key to resolving these problems. This consultation should be enacted when a mother is considering abandoning her child, when a child is found, when a child is adopted into a new family, and when the child becomes an adult. As one *sangoma* sagely advised me, 'It is the truth that sets you free.'

Material, financial, familial and psychological circumstances influence a mother in her decision to abandon a child. While abandonment implies cutting ties, for the mother sometimes this decision is about ensuring her own place within a family. The idea of losing family support or being abandoned by a boyfriend may lead a woman whose support structures are already thin to consider abandoning her child (Blackie 2017). While adoption implies being taken into a family, it does not guarantee the child a place in the family, or permanent inclusion. Both adoption and abandonment highlight the fragility of family bonds. As a result, many women use other strategies to maintain their families and keep their children.

The next case study (3.4) returns us to Soweto, where one in five households has no formal income. Many residents resort to informal ways of making ends meet, including selling sex, despite its being criminalised in South Africa. Sex workers face police harassment, violence and discrimination in their communities, exclusion from health services, and lack of access to justice in cases of physical and sexual assault. In this context of marginalisation and risk, a major reason that sex workers offered when describing their entry into the sex industry was caring for others (see also Walker 2017; Walker et al. 2017). As Susann Huschke describes in case study 3.4, many participants felt responsible for the lives, dreams and wellbeing of their children, younger siblings, parents, nieces and nephews, and sex work was a strategy that some women used to provide for and keep families together. Her engaged research in Soweto extended over 19 months between December 2015 and July 2017, during which time the women – Huschke and her interlocuters – worked together on artwork and narratives (Huschke 2017). As the participants recounted to Huschke, and illustrated through their own work, care for others was a source of pride, and their narratives of responsibility were a way of reclaiming a sense of moral and social worth in the face of stigmatisation and exclusion.

Case study 3.4

'I did well for my family'

Susann Huschke

> My name is Star. I am a 27-year-old mother of 3. I started doing sex work at the age of 16 when my older sister was very sick and needed money to go to doctors and traditional healers coz back then we were ignorant about HIV/AIDS. Life was so hard. I was in grade 10 then. My Mom and Dad were not working, so I had to do something to help. At that time the only option was to go to a tavern, and I knew boys who would offer me money in exchange, and yes, it was hard, but life went on.

Star is one of the sex workers who took part in Know My Story, a participatory arts-based project that formed part of the ethnographic study (Huschke 2017). In South Africa, both selling and buying sexual services is criminalised. Nevertheless, sex work constitutes an important informal livelihood strategy, particularly for working-class African women. The sex workers I spoke to started selling sex for various reasons, notably poverty and lack of other feasible employment opportunities. In total, 38 sex workers participated in this research: 34 were cis gender women, three identified as trans women and one as a gay man, reflecting the composition of the Soweto sex industry. The participants in this project either lived in one of the typical township 'matchbox houses', also known as RDP houses, built in rows like barracks, or in a backyard shack, built to accommodate extended families.

Only two participants had been able to access tertiary education, paying for the fees with a day job as peer educators in the local sex-worker health clinic. Many had not finished their matric (Grade 12 exams), often due to economic pressures, as education – including public primary education and public higher education – is fee based, and families also need to pay for school uniforms and school materials. Furthermore, public schools in predominantly African neighbourhoods offer poor-quality education – the lasting effects of the racially segregated school system under apartheid (Coetzee 2014). As a result, young African people continue to be disadvantaged in the shrinking labour market. Some participants had held jobs in the service sector, such as stacking boxes in supermarkets or selling fast food; others had never had formal employment; and a few had secured jobs as peer educators in a sex-worker health clinic.

What is love?

During apartheid, the South African economy centred on mining industries that needed large labour forces, triggering migration of African men from rural areas to mining towns such as Johannesburg and creating a dependence on wage labour. With the decline of these industries and the economic changes brought on by neoliberal policies of the post-apartheid governments, unemployment grew significantly, leading to the 'virtual ending of a "patriarchal bargain" in which men earned wages to provide housing and food for their families' (Hunter 2010: 62). Even so, the expectation remains that a man provide for his family, and participants in this study commonly expressed the hope of finding a reliable boyfriend who would provide for them and their children, ideally one who would be able to pay and marry them. Common descriptions of a good boyfriend focused on his ability 'to buy things' and 'take care of me and my children'.

This ideal crudely clashes with township life. Relationships are often not permanent, and marriage is very uncommon as few men can afford to pay *lobola*. Many of the sex-working mothers I spoke to were not in a relationship with the father(s) of their children anymore. None of the 34 women who took part in this research – aged between 22 and 45 years – was married. It was, however, common for women (and gay men) to have a boyfriend and a number of *makhwapheni* (translated by participants as 'side-dish', literally meaning 'under the armpit') (see Hunter 2010). For example, Lindiwe, a 22-year-old mother to a toddler, was torn between her love for the father of her son and her material needs, which led her to start a relationship with another man: 'This partner [the *makhwapheni*] gives me money. He's working and the father of my son is not working. I love him but the problem is he can't provide me with anything and the child and my mum – nobody is working at home. Sometimes you go to bed without eating.' The decision to sell sex to make a living needs to be understood in this context of unemployment, complex and fluid sexual relationships, gender norms that construct men as providers (see also McBride and Khumalo's case study 4.6), and the close connection between sex and money. Sex workers framed their choices as an expression of care and responsibility in the absence of viable alternatives.

Taking charge

Star's life story, introduced above, continues:

> Life was bad but I told myself all my life I have to fight to get money to
> help my sister to heal, to help my parents to eat, to help myself to live.
> While people call me *magosha* – whore – I would make myself strong so
> that my family could live. Hatred and discrimination is what I have come
> across since I was 16. At that age, I should be going to school, playing like
> other kids and treated like a child in my community but … things don't
> go as you expect them to. I grew up and thought to myself: it's hard, but I
> have to fight. No job, no money, that's not the life I am going to live.

Star asserts herself as a person with dignity and refuses to lose her sense of self-worth, as her community would have her do, over the fact that she has been selling sex to support herself and her family. Informal and criminalised ways of making money – including selling sex – were crucial for survival for many working-class African families. The average price for sex in Soweto's taverns and shebeens during the time of the research was around R50 (US$4), while sex workers working in hotels and upper-class bars in Soweto and other parts of Johannesburg may charge an hourly fee (for example R200 (US$16) or a fee per service (for example R150 (US$12) for vaginal sex). The income people generated with sex work varied greatly therefore: some research participants, working in hotels, earned R2 000 a week or more; others, typically from severely disadvantaged economic backgrounds, only made R200 in a week or sometimes nothing at all. For comparison, the average formal income per household in Johannesburg is R30 000 (US$2 200) per month for white residents and R5 600 (US$410) per month for Africans (City of Johannesburg 2012). In Soweto, people earned only R2 600 (US$208) per month on average. This income had to cover the costs of living for, on average, four people per household (City of Johannesburg 2005). A monthly income of as little as R500 made a significant difference to everyday living costs; an income of several thousand rands could help pay for school fees, house extensions, or medical costs.

In their written life stories, sex workers exemplified the relevance of sex work as a way of taking care of one's family and providing for basic human needs (and, one might argue, basic human rights) such as food, clothes and education. Amanda, a woman in her early forties who migrated to Soweto from the rural Eastern Cape, stressed how sex work enabled her to look after her two daughters, including paying the fees for her eldest to study for a college degree in law:

> I am a very protective mother. I have two beautiful girls; one is doing her
> first year in university, the other is still a baby. I love my babies so much.
> They are the reason I wake up every day. I am a proud mom; I did well for
> my family.

Similarly, Keletso, a woman in her early thirties, insisted on her identity as a responsible, caring mother:

> I am a girl from Limpopo who has three lovely boys. People fail to
> understand when I say I have three boys because they know I was
> pregnant once. But I adopted two. My first born I adopted him when my
> sister passed away. Last year, I adopted the child from my late friend Mary.
> We were like blood sisters and knew everything about each other. I am a
> single mother who goes all out for her children. Before you judge me know
> my story. I am a sex worker. What or who is a sex worker? A sex worker is
> a human being, a mother, and a person who has scars.

All the sex workers I worked with came from working-class African backgrounds, many from very economically disadvantaged families, but it would be deterministic to argue that economic deprivation 'forces' people into the sex industry.

Anti-sex-work lobbyists, generally white middle-class women, have for decades framed sex workers as victims without agency, in need of rescue (for example Jeffreys 1997). Globally, this has been strongly opposed by sex workers and their allies, who demand, for example, 'rights not rescue' and the decriminalisation of the sex industry (see Huschke 2016; Huschke & Dlamini 2017). Zenande, a participant in this study, eloquently put it this way: 'PITY – I cannot tolerate. CHARITY – I cannot live off! MY PRIDE – in making a living and being able to sustain myself and my family with a dream of one day returning to school to further my education.' Thus, while poverty is an important structural factor, the decision to sell sex to make a living is more complex. Not all poor women become sex workers. In fact, most do not.

When sex workers in Soweto discussed their lives and choices, love, responsibility and ambition emerged as key themes. The people I collaborated with felt responsible for the wellbeing of other people, and refused to give up hope to realise their own dreams of prosperity and happiness. They did not accept the place to which they were assigned by patriarchal norms, a racist economy and a stratified education system: at home, waiting for a male provider to bring a better life. What I view as courage and commitment, however, is often perceived as a disgrace by sex workers' families and communities, as I describe below.

Facing stigma

Sex work is everywhere a stigmatised income-generating strategy, although the form, texture and tone of the abuse and exclusion sex workers face vary depending on cultural context. In Soweto, contradictory moralities are attached to the omnipresent connection between sex and money (see also Hunter 2010). On the one hand, exchanging sex for money is a common and accepted practice; in relationships with boyfriends, *makhwapheni* and blessers (the local term for older 'sugar daddies'), it goes without saying that in return for money, drinks, food or other gifts, the male partner is entitled to sex. For Lihle, a woman in her mid-thirties, this social norm was reinforced by the aunt who raised her after the death of her mother and grandmother. Still in high school, Lihle started having sex for money: 'We would go on weekends from Friday then come back Sundays or Mondays. My aunt would never ask or shout at me as long as I brought her money and alcohol, she was OK.'

When Lihle entered into a relationship with an older man to whom she was not attracted, and who later abused her physically and sexually, her aunt focused on her contributions to the household: 'He took me for shopping, bought me clothes, toiletries etc. Then I introduced him to my aunt who welcomed him with open arms because she could see that since I was a responsible woman; I brought groceries home.'

Other sex workers made very similar points, reiterating that as long as one brings food or money home, no questions will be asked; it will be assumed that the material support is coming from a boyfriend or lover. Buhle is a 24-year-old sex-working mother of two children and breadwinner for her household, which included her mother, her two younger sisters and their two children. I asked her whether her family knew where the money she brought home came from (from selling sex in taverns). She responded: 'No. They think that I love going out with friends and I have this boyfriend of mine who has money.'

This was the common 'cover story' for sex workers who were the breadwinners for their families. Most sex workers worried that their families would find out that the money they earned came from clients, and not (multiple) boyfriends. However, the boundaries between clients and boyfriends were often blurred, and most sex workers who participated in this study have regular clients whom they consider friends, with whom they spend time talking, sharing meals and going out. The difference is not so much about what they do with each other, but how this is communicated or framed: with a client, payment is clearly expected in exchange for sex, whereas with a boyfriend or lover, there is generally no conversation about the nature of the relationship, despite the fact that the actual expectations (on both sides) might be similar: the male partner is expected to provide, and in return he is entitled to sex.

Despite similarities in the relationships between client and sex worker and those between boyfriend and girlfriend relationships, the former are highly stigmatised while the latter are not. A woman such as Lihle who brings home groceries that her blesser bought for her is considered to be a 'responsible woman'; if she buys groceries with money she earned as a sex worker, she is labelled a 'magosha'. The fundamental difference between these income-generating strategies is that a woman who relies on a boyfriend or lover to feed and clothe her and her family adheres to the patriarchal norm of the male provider; a sex worker earning her own money and taking the credit for it subverts this norm by claiming the role of the financially independent woman in control of her own life. When engaging in (morally acceptable) transactional sex, the woman remains the recipient of the man's care, whereas in (morally unacceptable) sex work, the woman is both breadwinner and provider. The interactions between sex workers and clients can, in many cases in South Africa, be read as expressions of patriarchal power dynamics, as radical feminists such as Carole Pateman (1999) have posited. However, the stigma attached to selling sex also rests on patriarchal norms that define men as providers and women as dependents. Trading sex for money is acceptable only if it does not rewrite gender norms and threaten men's position in society.

Heads held high

Out of fear of being judged, excluded or beaten, most sex workers who took part in this study kept their work a secret. Despite (or because of) the fact that they earned a living by working a job with many risks – including police violence, abuse from clients and exposure to sexually transmitted infections (STIs) – often they did not feel that they could claim acceptance, let alone respect, from their families and communities. For the sex workers who joined the participatory project that I facilitated, the key issue was to fight stigma and claim a sense of self-worth. How they told their stories expressed this tension between their embodied experiences of, on the one hand, patriarchal hierarchies, sexual double standards, and physical vulnerability to abusive and exploitative men, and, on the other, their own sometimes tender, sometimes angry, assertions of pride and defiance. They presented themselves as survivors, breadwinners, dreamers.

Meme – a woman in her mid-twenties, a mother of one and a student of social work – explained:

> Yes, I am a sex worker but then, sex work is only my profession, my source of income to earn a living. I have dreams, ambitions, responsibilities, and myself to look after. I have a son who is my everything. To me, he is the reason I wake up every day and go hustle to make ends meet for him. All I want for him is a proper life and good education. Dreams may seem shattered but nothing is impossible 'til it's done. I am struggling to pay for my tuition fees, thus my hustling does it for me. I still believe that some day, no matter how and when, I will hold that degree somehow. I am aiming for a brighter future for me and my family.

Pretty – orphan, rape survivor, mother and provider for her deceased sister's children and her elderly mother – said:

> I am a mother of a son, he is nine years old. He is a good son. He respects others. He likes school. And I have nephews that I have to take care of. If the child goes to school with an empty stomach what is he or she going to learn? Nothing, with an empty stomach! I am a hero because life was difficult when I grew up, but I didn't give up in life. Here I am.

And of course Star, who concluded her life story in this way:

> My community knew what I was doing but never accepted it 'cause they would talk about me when I passed through, saying ugly stuff. I had to stay strong. I succeeded. My sister got better and better. She is strong, healthy and beautiful now and she is the only family member that knows my story. Life has changed for the better.

In South Africa, the portrait of African youth is depressing. There are approximately 9.5 million young people 15–24 years of age; of that figure, 4.6 million are young women and girls (Stats SA 2019). According to the DoH's *National Adolescent and Youth Health Policy* (DoH et al. 2017), almost 2 000 young women and girls are infected with HIV every week. While the rate of teenaged pregnancy has steadily declined over the last two decades, the decrease is slower than expected (Ardington et al. 2012; Jewkes et al. 2010; Mkwanazi 2017). Gender-based violence and coerced sex are prevalent, as are transactional relationships (Leclerc-Madlala 2003; Russell et al. 2014). The level of youth unemployment is high and as already noted, many young people, especially women, drop out of school due to pregnancy and/or other reasons (DoH et al. 2017). Many young people who complete their schooling are unable to enter tertiary education due to rising costs, or to find a job due to the fierce competition for few jobs.[4] Young women face further difficulties due to a preference, by employers, for male employees. Education and health are key challenges in young people's lives. Although many young people live under challenging conditions, which are, in most instances, a result of a historical legacy, many try within such constraints to create opportunities to better their lives, and they fiercely defend their choices.

Case study 3.5, the final case study of this chapter, by Lebohang Masango, can be read alongside the experiences that young men growing up in townships face as described by Swartz's case study 4.2, for an understanding of comparative issues for young working-class men. It can also be read alongside Madhuha and Núñez Carrasco's case study 4.5, to compare self-care as enacted by older, rural men in Limpopo. Masango focuses on young women who use digital platforms to initiate intimate and/or sexual relationships, with money and sex forming the basis of the couple's transactions. Susann Huschke has already mentioned the role of the blesser, and in case study 3.5 Masango draws on her field research in Gauteng to focus on blesser–blessee relationships (Masango 2019). Such relationships may be somewhat disguised as 'age disparate' or 'intergenerational' (Leclerc-Madlala 2008) or explicitly included as a form of 'transactional sex' (Shefer et al. 2008), since the exchanges of money, gifts and sex are core features, and, often, strategies of subsistence (Bhana 2015; Hunter 2010; Selikow & Mbulaheni 2013; for a comparable example in Zimbabwe see Masvawure 2010). While the relationship may grow to be more than merely transactional, young women speak openly about their reasons for why money is important in the relationship. They also speak about the kinds of self-care they exercise to keep themselves safe from cyber and/or physical violence, and how they protect themselves from pregnancy or acquiring a sexually transmitted infection when they engage in sexual relationships with older men for money or gifts.

Case study 3.5

Tender blessing care

Lebohang Masango

In South Africa, the #blesser phenomenon began when young women posted photographs of their luxury goods and expensive holiday destinations on social media such as Twitter and Instagram with the caption #blessed. Through great public speculation on how these often unemployed or early-career women could afford such expensive lifestyles, the hashtag gradually came to indicate a secret 'sugar daddy' relationship between an older, and often married, man (#blesser) and a young woman (#blessee).

A glance at the type of imagery that populates the #blessed hashtag reveals that a substantial factor distinguishes #blessed from other compensated relationships. Firstly, conspicuous consumption – not economic subsistence – is central to #blesser relationships; secondly, young women engage in these relationships in order to supplement their already consumerist, middle-class lifestyles. Although the differences are not vast, these two points are important; they allow the possibility of interrogating the lives of middle-class youth and emerging postfeminist and neoliberal feminist subjectivities through young women's engagement in social media communities.

The controversy generated by #blessed gained momentum beyond mobile phones and computer screens, and enjoyed media attention on prime-time talk-radio shows (for example, *The Eusebius McKaiser Show* on Radio 702) and television programmes (for example, the investigative current affairs programme *Checkpoint*). This momentum re-energised public conversations about sexuality, health, women's agency and conceptions of love. However, it quickly devolved into 'slut-shaming' and the moral reproach of young women, contrasting with the silence around the men who enabled these relationships. The public outcry against blessees was fuelled by three public panics, mainly: health, safety and moral questions equating #blessees to sex workers. I address each of these concerns below.

Bohlale was a 20-year-old student of engineering at the University of the Witwatersrand, who lived in 'res' (student accommodation). Unlimited access to Wi-Fi, and boredom between lectures and homework, led her to venture beyond using her mobile phone for common social media such as Twitter, Facebook and Tumblr – platforms that encourage the uploading of user-generated media content and facilitate communication within one's network. Bohlale is a self-proclaimed 'sugar baby', or professional girlfriend, who began to experiment with online dating platforms such as Tinder and Seeking Arrangement in order to receive an allowance from her romantic relationships. But she neither dates men *for* money, nor is she a sex worker. Rather, her romantic relationships are ordinary couplings, except that she expects to be monetarily compensated for her time, energy and emotion. Here, her labour refers to the practical yet gendered aspects of emotional care, such as being a good listener, offering solutions to problems, and fostering a space of mutual vulnerability and trust within the relationship. Her experiences provide insights to challenge the dominant narratives around such compensated relationships.

We are five days into the new year and although the university will remain closed until February, the campus is full of students making use of the library and the different administration facilities for registration. The sky is clear and blue, yet the air is unnervingly hot, with the kind of sunlight that forces everyone into spots of shade for relief. Bohlale and I are sitting cross-legged on the lawns in front of the library. She's dressed in a brown coat with long black slacks, and she is sipping on coffee. It makes sense; it's the kind of outfit that's necessary for braving Wits's perennially cold exam halls.

Bohlale describes herself as a 'sugar baby', a phrase she encountered on Tumblr where she became a part of 'sugar baby Tumblr', the online community of mostly American sex workers and professional girlfriends who use the blogging platform to give each other advice, and share experiences and survival strategies on how to navigate their often dangerous daily interactions with men. Online anonymity and the inability to verify identities and information, coupled with the offline risks of physical and sexual abuse, are some of the ways in which sugar babies are specifically endangered.

Bohlale also uses Seeking Arrangement, a dating portal for self-proclaimed sugar daddies seeking young, college-educated young women. The website invites men to pay for membership and specify their financial income in order to facilitate 'arrangements' or compensated relationships. This particular figure of the sugar daddy is closely aligned to what is also referred to as a blesser.

Sexual health

In discussing her latest arrangement, which arose from Curious Cat, a Twitter-affiliated platform, Bohlale offered insight into her sexual-health practices:

> He was like, 'Look, I don't expect you to be monogamous or anything, that doesn't really make sense with our situation.' We were having a full disclosure thing, where if you have a partner you disclose and he's also really adamant about not having kids. I thought I was serious about that shit – he's *serious* about that shit. He's like, 'I'm gonna get a vasectomy.' Some of the finances he provides were like, 'Do you wanna get birth control? Do you need anything?' Before we were going on our Stellenbosch trip, I was telling him that I wanna get a full STI screening but they're so expensive and he's like, 'Look, I know a place and I can book an appointment for you with the guy I went to and I'll take care of it

because the reason why you're doing this anyway is for me.' The last time I'd taken a full STI screening was last year and I like to make it a yearly thing. Before our first date, he'd already given me his and he was just putting it out there. I think that's why I was like, 'Yay! Viva!' when we met the first time ...

It's borderline paranoia but I'm really serious about three things: the health thing, like if someone won't give me their HIV results or STI results then I'm like, 'Not gonna work.' Anyone that's against using protection for any reason, I'm like, 'No that's not gonna work.' I'm really strict on the consent thing because I try – and this is why I think ... I lose out on a lot of guys because people think that the 'exchange' takes away the consent: so if I give you R3 000, I can do whatever I want to you for the weekend? *No,* no, no, no. That's not the deal. So I'm really clear about that. If it seems like the person isn't grasping what I'm saying or I sense the entitlement then I'm like, 'You know what? I appreciate that we've gotten this far in our conversation but I don't think you're the guy for me and it's not gonna work.'

Bohlale's recounting of her talk with her partner shows that multiple sexual partners are likely. She tells of how her partner is honest and forthcoming about his STI test results, and is willing to pay for her screening and contraceptives. She later emphasises the importance of her sexual health: she insists on condom use and she does not engage in sex until a partner discloses his STI test results. Her insistence on consent is at the centre of the relationship, and she engages in fewer relationships because potential partners are dissuaded by her stance. Bohlale terminates relationships if her partners do not comply with her standards.

Prevailing stereotypes around compensated relationships as a danger to young women's sexual health and agency are reinforced by the current public-health discourse that implicates young women in South Africa's rising statistics on HIV infections (Gouws & Williams 2016; Shisana et al. 2014). Health experts assert that young women 15–24 years of age are highly susceptible to HIV exposure through sexual relationships with older men due to asymmetries of power related to age, financial status and social capital; these factors make it difficult to negotiate condom use and other safe-sex practices (Leclerc-Madlala 2008). However, Bohlale demonstrates that cautionary care in the form of safe sexual-health practices can be, although it is not always, exercised in relationships where the disparities of power are pronounced, and can include disengaging if they are a threat to one's agency.

Online and offline safety

Bohlale's experiences as a sugar baby have made her conscious of her personal security while using social media. Her interaction with her community of peers on Tumblr, and on a newer social network called Peach, have equipped her with strategies to navigate her relationships, which are usually initiated online with strangers. A consistent risk for blessees is the threat of predatory men who target professional girlfriends and sex workers to manipulate them, threatening to expose their personal information and deceive them by cheating them of the money agreed upon in their arrangement. A former boyfriend managed to learn Bohlale's real name, and had used it to taunt her into granting him a date. Bohlale explains various strategies she has developed:

> I have an entire business email now because I realised that you don't use your real email for these things … I swear, I even ended up deactivating Facebook and for Tinder, I ended up making a decoy Facebook – that was a suggestion from the girls on Peach. They're like, 'Don't worry. This happens sometimes', 'cause some of the girls are escorts and protecting their identity is more high stakes, and they're like, 'Just block him, ignore him, don't answer him, don't get into the threats and the mind games. Just leave it. Make sure that everything of yours is protected.' I immediately deactivated my Facebook and everything else with my government name. I don't have a LinkedIn and stuff. I did the whole thing where you Google yourself and you make sure that you can't find yourself anywhere. That was pretty much it … No, don't use your real email. Make a proper, proper email and use an alias and you can use that alias for anything you want. What shows up on my Tinder now is my alias, which is close enough to my name so if anyone ever finds my name I say, 'I wasn't lying though, and it's my middle name or my nickname.' I made an alias with a completely fake surname though … the one thing that I don't do is use pictures posted on any other social media for Tinder.

Currently, users of social media services and websites on the internet have their personal information secured through logging in processes that include email address and user name authentication. Some social media, such as Tinder, also require users to sign up with their Facebook profile to confirm some basic personal details and create matches among potential dates that are dependent on location, age and interests.

In an act of goodwill towards her followers, some of whom may be young women who are pursuing a similar lifestyle to hers, Bohlale created a Twitter thread related to the precautions that are necessary when shifting from online texting and emailing to offline, in-person interactions. Her thread includes suggestions about reverse searching of images to determine identity, sharing a date's personal details with a trusted contact, not meeting for the first time in a dark and loud venue, and, finally, undertaking a name search on the university database if a person claims to be at the same institution.

Another concern regarding young women who are engaged in compensated relationships is their personal safety. In an 2017 article on the IOL news website, Sonke Gender Justice spokesperson Karen Robertson is reported as stating that although the concept of revenge porn (publishing a person's sexually explicit imagery without consent) has only recently emerged with the rise of social media, it is an extension of rape culture and objectifies women.[5] Bohlale avoids compromising situations that could result in access to explicit material, and she ensures that measures for basic security are well implemented. She demonstrates a great deal of care by engaging in an online community that offers helpful safety and survival strategies and, in turn, she shares that knowledge with others.

Fuck you money

Bohlale's speaks of 'fuck you money' – the money she receives from compensated relationships that she uses to increase her independence *from* men. The intersection of her dating lifestyle, her feminist stance and the role of money is expressed as a postfeminist sensibility (Gill 2007). In our continued conversation, Bohlale articulated this relationship at length:

My feminism actually demands that I be like this and I date in this kind of way ... money is empowering to women. If I have fuck you money, it gives me independence; it gives me the ability to leave you whenever I want to ... money is power and money is independence. The one thing that a lot of sex workers say, and it makes so much sense, is the fact that people villainise sex work because they're like: 'Oh my gosh, you're using your body and it's degrading and there's no dignity it ... ' This is the one argument that I really despise, they say that women are driven into sex work because they don't have money, but everyone is driven into every kind of work because they don't have money, especially in South Africa. People don't care about that primarily because it's not deemed as sexually deviant, the people that do it are not usually women and it's been male labourers who have been farmers ... And also, capitalism relies on people making money for other people and the deviance in sex work has always been that ... independent sex workers make money for themselves.

The other angle that I always like to look from is that as a woman, just by existing, I am immediately sexually objectified. I am a sexual object and I'm going to do all of this labour regardless of whether I charge for it or not. People are making money off me ... In a lot of social spaces actually: the dating scene, when you go out and the guy is like, 'I'll pay to take a girl out to dinner but I won't give her money directly.' Why? He feels more comfortable giving the establishment money than giving you money ... He expects you to do sexual labour after that but you did not benefit from that, I mean, you ate a frickin' croissant and some snails or whatever and that's not really beneficial to you. So for me, the way that it ties into my feminism is that it's political in terms of the larger economic theme of the exchange of money directly between working-class women and upper-class men. I think that's the one thing that sex work is able to do that no other sector can do …

Money buys me experiences, it frees up my time, it makes living in this city and being a student so much better … people like to ignore that in a capitalist society, money buys you freedom – that's why everyone works because we want more freedom, we want more time to spend with our families, we want more money to give to the ones we love and be able to provide.

Bohlale's engagement in compensated relationships is informed by her feminist beliefs and is ultimately an act of great self-care. At the intersection of capitalism and robust social-media consumption, young women, like Bohlale, are identifying opportunities to engage romantically with men in ways that strictly prioritise themselves. At one end of the spectrum, there is #FeesMustFall, which has exposed South African society to the racialised and gendered financial, social and psychological burdens of acquiring higher education for the majority of young people in the country. At the other end, there is #MenAreTrash, an ongoing public conversation about men perpetrating gender-based violence in South Africa. Between these two powerful hashtag movements, young women are choosing to shun utopian ideals of love in favour of more pragmatic approaches that explicitly take account of their wellbeing and the socioeconomic climate. Despite public knowledge of risks associated with intergenerational sexual relationships and the potential harms of initiating intimate relationships with strangers from the internet, young women are using social media as a solution. Their online communities of support and their shrewd realism lead them to make empowering life decisions.

Poor individuals, families and households have all found ways to provide care and support each other. As we have demonstrated, fathers do help with childcare and support childcare decisions, and family members care for children other than their own, when fathers do not (and cannot) provide financial help. Some women take on sex work; others are given cash and gifts for sex within affectionate relationships. Some decisions are pragmatic and are based on available resources and space; others are future looking and require short-term sacrifices to achieve a better life in the future. As we have shown, family members often set aside their own aspirations to endure uncertainty, even risking violence and arrest to keep their family together. One of the dominant themes associated with keeping families together is 'sacrifice'. Women more than men are likely to put their lives on hold and sacrifice their own aspirations for the wellbeing of others.

In this chapter, we have shown that women desire to be seen as 'good' mothers and make decisions in this context, including in relation to feeding and care, and to who takes on everyday care. In resource-poor communities, finding ways to earn respectability and to be seen as a good mother is important (Blake 2017; Mkhwanazi & Bhana 2017). The desire to be seen as a good mother is manipulated by the state, which uses it as an entry point to influence how women care for their children. An act such as infant feeding thus becomes political, as well as, for women, a way to communicate their identity and medical biography.

There are many different and competing ideas about what constitutes 'good' mothering, a 'good' woman, a 'good' citizen. Ideas about the 'good' mothering and good sexual behaviour are often political and moral. The state often aims to promote a particular agenda which, in the case of mothering, may be underpinned by particular ideas about the body and the ideal circumstances for human development. Discourses of 'good' are also ways of reproducing the status quo, and statements about being a good mother and raising a child are commonly couched in terms of adhering to 'tradition' or 'culture'. In the case of both reproduction and sexuality, blame is typically placed on particular individuals and families – poor African women especially – so removing the responsibility of the state to provide conditions that could enable families to stay together and for mothers to better protect their children.

Notes

1   Child Welfare South Africa, Cape Town and Johannesburg, estimate child abandonment 2009/2010 at over 3 500 babies and children, *Weekend Post,* 27 August 2010.

2   A baby safe is a modern-day version of the eighteenth-century 'foundling wheel', where a baby is placed in a safe constructed in the wall of a place of safety to allow mothers to abandon their child anonymously.

3   Jabulani Mphalal, KZN Commissioner for Traditional Leadership Disputes and Crimes, 21 February 2014, quoted in 'African ancestral beliefs make baby abandonment preferable to adoption', *All4Women,* 28 May 2014. Accessed 10 November 2019, https://www.all4women. co.za/206149/news/african-ancestral-beliefs-make-baby-abandonment-preferable-to-adoption

4   Omarjee L, Unemployment rate drops 26.7%, *Fin24,* 13 February 2018.

5   Cloete N, 'Revenge porn, slut shaming implicated in rape', *IOL,* 9 July 2017. Accessed November 2019, https://www.iol.co.za/news/south-africa/western-cape/revenge-porn-slut-shaming-implicated-in-rape-10202945

4 *How men care*

Lenore Manderson and Nolwazi Mkhwanazi

In contemporary South Africa, both customary and civil marriage has declined. While some couples may intend to marry and initiate *lobola* payments, unemployment and poverty make this kind of marriage for many a mere dream. Historically, decisions about the care of children born to parents who are not married were governed by certain codes of conduct. Firstly, the pregnant woman's family approached the family of the genitor to report the pregnancy. Following that, if the pregnancy was acknowledged and paternity accepted, then a discussion about the payment of *inhlawulo* ensured (see Chapter 1 for a discussion of *inhlawulo*). Once a price was agreed on, then the payment – *inhlawulo* – was made, and only after the full payment was concluded was the child seen as belonging to the patrilineal lineage. Paying damages did not mean that at a later stage the parents of the child were obliged to marry, but it did incorporate the child into the patrilineage; as was explained in the previous chapter and particularly in Deirdre Blackie's case study (3.3), this is regarded as very important. But not being in a legal union with the mother of one's child, and not having legal ties to one's child, puts men in a precarious position in relation to children. In this chapter, we turn to men's aspirations, expectations and experiences of care of intimate partners and children.

Historically, during colonial rule and under the apartheid state, stable heterosexual relationships were largely rendered impossible, as men from rural areas were recruited to work firstly in mines and secondly as wage labour for expanding infrastructure, industry and urban development. While women may have aspired to live in family units, and most women and men held (and still hold) personal beliefs consistent with heteronormativity, historically and in the present, many families have consisted of women and children, or of women, children, and patrilines. Households and families are centred on women of different generations and relationships with each other, as has already been illustrated in relation to infants, household economies and domestic labour, childcare and support, household health and intimate care, are very much women's work.

Given that this is the case, for practical and ideological reasons men have been treated as ancillary to reproduction resulting in their distance from biological reproduction, the sustainment of households and the bringing up of children. Yet this overlooks the significance of having families, and the ideal of 'the family', for many men. In this context, patrilineal kinship structure supports a strong desire that lineage be maintained, and property and children protected through marriage (customary or other), even if its formal acknowledgement is deferred to some time in the future. Moreover, men see the fulfilment of their roles as husbands and fathers to be consistent with cultural values around masculinity and manliness, as has been illustrated recurrently (Jewkes et al. 2015; Morrell et al. 2012). Ideals of maleness, built on notions of men's physical and structural superiority, link political, economic and sexual power and the exercise of privilege. Former president Jacob Zuma embodied and enacted these notions of hegemonic masculinity as a traditional patriarch and polygamist (Hunter 2010). The concept of hegemonic masculinities helps explain gendered ideals linked to masculinities that are widely held and reproduced in society.

Hegemonic masculinity operates in ways that are not particular to all African men, nor to Zulu and Xhosa men. Rather, across communities, particularly among working-class men, common ideas are held about men's positioning in relation to women, and there continue to be sharp distinctions between men and women in terms of access to education, employment, pay and advancement, personal safety and life choices. Adherence to hegemonic masculinity ideas works to reinforce and reproduce these distinctions. Gender theory and theories of hegemonic masculinity propose that how any man identifies, relates and behaves as a man is strongly influenced by prevailing cultural norms of masculinity, and this provides a pathway to reduce violence. In theory, men can personally and collectively choose to challenge cultural norms.

We turn now to how men are involved in decisions about retaining a pregnancy, in supporting a partner, and in contributing to parenting and creating a family, and to providing care and physical and economic support. Men's involvement in family life occurs in the context of chronic unemployment, in rural South Africa especially. The growing service sector – entertainment, tourism, retail and offices – has created more jobs for young women than men (Collinson et al. 2016), leaving rural men especially with the time, if not motivation, to contribute to domestic production and caregiving. But men do not necessarily resist such contributions to the home, and for some the birth of an infant is profound and life changing.

Case study 4.1, by Nozipho Mvune and Deevia Bhana, is set in rural KwaZulu-Natal and is based on qualitative research conducted by Mvune and her colleagues in Illovo in the rural Ugu District (see Mvune et al. 2019 for a description of the research methods). The research involved interviews with 30 teenage fathers. With a few exceptions, teenage fathers are largely invisible from the literature on teenage parents. However the lives of young fathers, and those of their partners, detour – and may be transformed – as a result of pregnancy and the birth of a child, as is the case for Sandile, the young man whose story the case study tells.

Case study 4.1

Sandile's story

Nozipho Mvune and Deevia Bhana

Sandile, who is 18 years old, shares the last encounter he had with his biological father, a 'stranger', on his deathbed:

> He told us all the terrible things that he had said to us in the past like we can starve … he didn't care, he told us that. And on his last day he begged us to forgive him. He looked sad, he actually had tears – you can imagine tears of an old man.

Sandile's story continues: his stepfather took over the role of father and supported Sandile and his siblings. In 2014, Sandile's stepfather died of tuberculosis, and Sandile spoke of the pain he felt and his deep sense of powerlessness at this time. His mother was the sole provider, relying on the Child Support Grant (CSG). When he turned 18 years old, Sandile's CSG benefit was terminated, but his mother continues to collect the grant for his three younger siblings and gets some help from an older relative.

A female-headed household in poverty, a household's reliance on CSG, and an absent father who does not provide any care (financial or otherwise): these are not unusual in impoverished African households (Richter et al. 2010; see also Richter & Morrell 2006). Owing to high rates of unemployment, many South African fathers are unable to pay either *inhlawulo* and/or *lobola*; as was explained in the previous chapters, inability to pay *inhlawulo* may rob a father of an opportunity to be part of his child's life. Dominant hegemonic notions of masculinity – often associated with drugs, alcohol abuse and multiple partners – all impact on young men (Mvune et al. 2019). Yet, as we describe, for Sandile, the path to becoming a father provided him with moments of reflection, allowing him to consider responsibility and renewed forms of power that could lead to changing masculinities.

Power and playboys

Growing up was not easy for Sandile:

> As a boy, I did all the bad things. At Grade 6 I started smoking cigarettes, moved to alcohol and dagga [marijuana] at Grade 7. I would save R5 each day so that on Friday I would have R35. We would put our monies together with my friends and buy a bottle of brandy. I think it's because of the friends that I had; *ja* [yes] we influenced each other to do those things. We would drink during [the school] break and smoke. After break, we would come back drunk and disturb classes. I think it was bad influence from friends. We would arrive late at school and sometimes bunk classes.

> When I was drunk I would feel good; alcohol made me feel like a different
> person, a person who is happy.

Through alcohol and drugs, Sandile was able to express power, derive pleasure,
work against the misery and drudgery of poverty, and gain power within his
group of friends. He had multiple girlfriends and his peer group called themselves
playboys:

> I was good when it comes to *ukweshela* [courting]. I was never turned
> down by a girl. So, I just couldn't wait to pass Grade 7 and come to high
> school. We were a group of nine friends; eight of us passed Grade 7 – only
> one failed. When we came to high school to do Grade 8, we gave our
> group a name; we called ourselves 'playboys'. We would sit together during
> break and eat cakes and cold drinks. We would ask any boy to go and call
> a child [girl] for us and he would go and return with that child. It was
> about showing off that *sibanibani uyayibamba le ngane* [so and so is in a
> relationship with this child], she belongs to him. Even when I was doing
> Grade 8 I had a girlfriend doing Grade 12.

The term 'playboy' – used for a man with multiple girlfriends – is not unusual
in rural KwaZulu-Natal. One older participant who took part in Mark Hunter's
(2010) study defined a 'playboy' as *isoka lamanyala* (a dirty *isoka*), a man with
many girlfriends without intention to marry any of them.

Sandile's aim as a playboy was to show off and earn the respect of his peers. Then
in 2015 he met Ntobe, who was 18 years old and studying in Grade 10. Sandile
was 17, and in the same class. He said that Ntobe was the most brilliant learner in
class, and she would do homework for both of them. Unlike other girls who saw
nothing wrong in sharing their playboy boyfriends (Bhana & Anderson 2013),
Ntobe would fight with any girl interested in a relationship with Sandile. Their
relationship was volatile:

> One night we had a big fight with Ntobe when she was visiting; she woke
> up in the middle of the night whilst I was sleeping. I saw her heating a
> spoon over the burning stove. She was crying saying she wants to burn
> my face so that I become less attractive to the other girlfriends. It was a
> big fight; I woke up and fought back, trying very hard to protect my face.
> My mother woke up because of the noise because we were both crying.
> She took Ntobe to sleep with her and I went back to my room. Luckily, I
> blocked the spoon with my hand and I only got a small scratch.

As was also noted in Chapter 2, many teenage heterosexual relationships are
imbued with gender-based violence (see also Russell et al. 2014). In some
instances, although not all, such violence is viewed as a sign of love and
commitment (Wood et al. 2008). Sandile's mother supported their relationship
and advised them to use protection. But Ntobe was already pregnant. Sandile

insisted he always had condoms and had protected sex, and Ntobe would insist 'no condom, no sex'. However:

> One day after having sex we saw that the condom was missing, we really got worried cos when we started I was wearing it. We found it inside Ntobe (in her vagina), so we don't know what happened … One night I visited her and when her parents were asleep, she allowed me to sneak into her bedroom and that night we had no protection … As a boyfriend, it's my duty to provide CDs [condoms] … we continued using condoms but sometimes we would have sex without protection.

Pregnancy

Ntobe became pregnant as a result of the inconsistent and incorrect use of condoms:

> One day she told me that she doesn't feel well. She said she has nausea; she feels sleepy and tired all the time. She said she suspects that she may be pregnant. So, she asked her friend to accompany her to the clinic and the nurses confirmed that she was pregnant. We just didn't know what to do, we were so afraid of what our parents would say. It was a very difficult time … we decided that we were not going to tell anyone until the pregnancy start showing. Only our close friends knew.

However, Ntobe did not carry the pregnancy to full term; she had a miscarriage at three months. When the local clinic referred Ntobe to hospital for a curette to 'clean out her womb', Sandile's mother went with her, providing both physical and emotional support. After the miscarriage, Ntobe and Sandile no longer used a condom or any other form of contraceptive. Two months after the miscarriage, Ntobe was pregnant again.

> We continued with our relationship. We were no longer using protection. After some time, she told me that she was pregnant again. The miscarriage was some time in June (2015), and she found out about the second pregnancy in August. My mother suspected that Ntobe was pregnant and asked her; she denied it, she just lied. My grandmother from Umlazi phoned my mother to say she was having strange dreams that someone was pregnant. My mother called both of us and asked if Ntobe was pregnant. We denied it until Ntobe started crying and admitted that she was pregnant.

Despite not using protection, Sandile insisted that the second pregnancy was not planned, and they were shocked. Sandile's mother told him to drop out of school and to find a job in order to provide for his child and assume his new role as a father.

My mother took me to another room and spoke strongly to me, telling me that I have to drop out of school to go and work for the baby now that I am a man. I managed to find a temporary job where I was helping one guy who is a local builder. I worked for him during weekends and school holidays and he paid me R100 each day. I spent it all on Ntobe's needs, like paying for her transport to the clinic. I stopped smoking and drinking in 2015; I just had to grow up. I spent every cent I had on Ntobe.

Being there for each other

Sandile made every effort to provide for Ntobe, taking on temporary jobs on weekends and during holidays and so meeting the socially set standards of masculinity. In addition, he found other ways to provide Ntobe with care and support, including academic support when she couldn't come to school:

She [Ntobe] was very brave; she came to school with her big tummy. She didn't care who said what. When exams for first term [2016] started, she was highly pregnant and only managed to write two subjects, then went to deliver the baby, our baby boy. When she was away, I would communicate with our school LSA [Learner Support Agent], who would give me some schoolwork from subject teachers, especially assessment tasks to pass on to Ntobe. Ntobe would do the [assessment] tasks and give them to me, so that I give them to the LSA, who would then forward them to the different subject teachers. This really helped Ntobe to have some marks in her subjects; but not all teachers gave the LSA the work.

Such stories of caring teenage fathers are often untold. Sandile was determined to be a supportive and caring father, to provide Ntobe and their child with a different experience from his own. The academic support that Sandile gave Ntobe, together with the LSA, enabled her to make a smooth re-entry to school. As Sandile explained, the LSA helps learners with problems that disturb learning, including linking the learner with social workers, referring the learner to the health clinic, and in other ways working with young pregnant women to ensure that they resume school after delivery. Both Sandile and Ntobe would talk to the LSA, although this was unusual:

Usually, it's pregnant girls or girls who have become mothers who go and talk to the LSA. Boys don't want the whole school to know that they have become fathers; most of them prefer to keep it a secret. So, I think that's why they [teenage fathers] don't want to be seen talking to the LSA. But, I'm telling you man, there are so many of us who are fathers here [at school]; we know each other and we protect each other's secret. When teachers get to know your story that you have become a father, it's like they want the whole world to know.

Stigma and shame prevent teenage fathers from getting support to help them negotiate fatherhood and schooling. Sandile continued, giving us an account of the day that his child was born:

> I was away with my school soccer team when my mother phoned me to tell me that Ntobe is in labour. She told me that she [my mother] had hired a car to take her [Ntobe] to the hospital. Around 8 p.m. my mother called me to say Ntobe has been taken to hospital. The following day around 8 in the morning my mother phoned me again and told me that I was a father to a baby boy.
>
> It was a great shock. I just cried and couldn't explain to my teammates … I think it was because I was very happy. I ended up telling teachers that I have just become a father – they couldn't believe it. I showed them the picture that my mother had sent via WhatsApp. I was very happy about becoming a father. As a result, that day I had a very good game; I managed to focus knowing that Ntobe and the baby were fine. After being told that I had become a father; I even ignored the girlfriends from other schools that I had found at a hotel where we were staying. My mother phoned me again to tell me that we can go together to the hospital the following day if I wanted to see the baby.

So Sandile shared his news with his teachers, despite the general expectation that boys and men should 'bury their emotions' (Kaufman 1993: 61). Sandile also told us about the relationship that he has with his son, Ayanda:

> My mother stays with our baby. I am saving every cent that I get for him and his mother. Whenever I look at him, it's like I see myself, he has my looks. He is very handsome. He has a beautiful smile like his mother. When my mother is busy with some of her duties, I hold Ayanda, tell him stories until he falls asleep … he sleeps with my mother but I also help, like making his bottle. It feels good to know that I get to see and spend time with him every day. Ntobe comes over to see him during the weekend but sometimes comes and spends time with him in the middle of the week and we go to school together. We never miss a day at school; we are always there for each other.

The above quotation points to a caring father who is actively involved with his infant and supporting his partner. Becoming a father provided Sandile with an opportunity to develop an alternative form of masculinity (Chili & Maharaj 2015) to using drugs, alcohol and having multiple partners. At the same time, despite his pride in becoming a father, Sandile's life was not without hardship:

> Things have changed now that I have a baby. My mother is spending money on the baby, like in December she didn't buy me new clothes and didn't give me any money. She told me that it's either me or the baby. It's

> very hard having a baby whilst you are still a child yourself. So, I am sure
> that it is going to take us a very long time before we think of another baby.
> We are both focusing on our education.

Sandile's story sheds light on the complexities surrounding teenage sexuality, especially in areas like rural KwaZulu-Natal, where there are especially high levels of poverty. In such contexts, teenagers engage in practices such as using drugs and alcohol, and have multiple intimate partners, practices that produce power but also risk (Mvune et al. 2019). This includes unplanned parenthood. Dominant masculine norms are reproduced as Sandile works to provide for his baby and girlfriend, but he provided academic as well as material support for his girlfriend and actively helped to care for his infant son. In contrast to his father, Sandile wants to be involved. While such masculinity is invested in dominant notions of provider status, it is also deeply caring.

Until the publication of *Teenage Tata: Voices of Young Fathers in South Africa* (Swartz & Bhana 2009), young fathers were largely ignored in the literature on early parenthood. The focus was almost exclusively on young mothers, partly because, in the past, a large number of the genitors of the children of teenage mothers denied paternity. For some, this denial was to do with poverty and fathers being unable (or unwilling) to support the upbringing of a child, or distrusting the mother's allegations of paternity. Hence they played no role in the care of the child, either by choice or by convention. Teenage mothers thus often relied on their own family, and so children born to teenage mothers were raised in matrifocal families.

In the last two decades, researchers have begun to write about the acknowledgement of paternity and the desire of men, especially young fathers, to be involved in their children's lives (Bhana & Nkani 2014; Chili & Maharaj 2015; Mvune et al. 2019). In contemporary African families, the decision about the involvement of paternal kin in caring for children of unwed mothers does not lie with the young mother or the young father, but rather with elder kinswomen (Mkhwanazi 2017; Nkani 2017). Where paternity was denied, the mother and her kin were often left to care for the child without patrilineal support, but the acknowledgement of paternity through the payment of damages allowed for paternal kin to care for the child (Mkhwanazi & Block 2016). Now, however, young men are accepting paternity even when they cannot pay damages. Some families accept the father's willingness to be involved in the care of the child despite his not having paid *inhlawulo*; others restrict the father's access to the child until he has done so (Nkani 2017; Mkhwanazi's case study 2.1; Pillay's case study 3.2).

In case study 4.2, we move from rural KwaZulu-Natal to an urban township in the Western Cape, and to Luyanda, a young man who, like Sandile, is still in school. The case study draws on data collected by Alison Swartz during long-term ethnographic fieldwork in Khayelitsha. This fieldwork began at the end of 2009 and remains ongoing. Luyanda's adolescence was marked by drug-taking and antisocial behaviour. Like Sandile in case study 4.1, Luyanda experienced his girlfriend's pregnancy and the birth of their infant as a turning point to perform a new type of masculinity, one that allowed him to demonstrate his virility and fertility, his responsibility towards his infant daughter, and his commitment – at least in the short term – to the mother of his daughter. In both cases, the infants were cared for by their paternal grandmothers; in this way, older women protect and support the young men, as well as young women, from potential defeat by the burdens of everyday caregiving and the search for sufficient income.

Case study 4.2

Saving face

Alison Swartz

Researchers have challenged depictions of linear and universal life-course transitions by highlighting the fact that such transitions are often partial, uneven and under threat (Johnson-Hanks 2002). Young people coming of age in township contexts like Khayelitsha are forced to negotiate income poverty, inadequate education and lack of access to employment. In Town Two, a neighbourhood of Khayelitsha, opportunities are often limited.

In this case study, I explore how one young man, Luyanda, attempted to navigate towards adulthood in the context of socioeconomic marginalisation. To make this transition, he used his performance of gender identity, sexual partnerships and early parenthood, while grappling with his own and others' expectations of him.

I met Luyanda in 2013 through a local pastor, who had been centrally involved in church-related work to try to encourage young men like Luyanda to end their participation in gang-related activity. Luyanda's smile and shoulders were equally broad. He played soccer and was captain of a local team. He wore clothing identified by athletic and outdoor brands. Luyanda lived in a *hokkie* (shack) at the back of his mother's three-roomed RDP house in Town Two. She was the sole income earner for the household, which included Luyanda, his older brother and girlfriend, an uncle and a few young children. Luyanda's mother experienced 'a lot of stress' to stretch as far as possible her modest salary from her employment at a supermarket.

When we met, Luyanda was an identified member of the church and had been through Xhosa initiation. He was no longer a gang member, but at the height of his involvement with the 'Hated But Respected' (HBR) gang in Town Two, he and his friends used to steal and smoke. He never smoked *tik* (methamphetamine), he said, but he did smoke cigarettes and marijuana. He still does, although he tries to disguise this. When he spoke about the violence of the past, it was with a combination of pride and shame. Several stories centred on his need to defend HBR territory and the honour of fellow gang members; at times though, he looked embarrassed by their violence.

Unlike several friends and fellow gang members expelled from local schools in Khayelitsha, Luyanda completed high school. In his final year, however, just before he began his matric exams, his girlfriend Andiswa told him that she was pregnant. Luyanda – unlike others, including friends, who denied paternity – said that he had planned the child and explained to Andiswa his intentions; before marrying, he wanted to 'check' how they managed having a child together. Luyanda was adamant that Andiswa was having his child, and that he wanted to support both her and her baby. With her pregnancy, Andiswa dropped out of school in Grade 10, and she did not return after their daughter was born. Luyanda was increasingly worried about not having work, because he said he needed to provide for Andiswa and their daughter. Over the next year and a half, he took on poorly paid contract jobs as a labourer with building or landscaping companies that paid him just R100 for a full day of work. He would often return home tired and dejected.

The next time I saw Luyanda, he had a sizable gash on the side of his face. The wound pulled at the right-hand corner of his mouth, and he was missing one front tooth and half of another. He had been hit in the face by a brick thrown by a boy aiming for a rival gang member. In trying to stop the fight, Luyanda had been caught in it.

Over time the wound healed, but Luyanda's smile was permanently changed. Whereas before he would greet people with his warm, crooked grin, his lips now remained tightly closed. Luyanda worried that he was earning so little money, and he applied for better-paying jobs. In two consecutive job interviews, he was told that he would have been offered the job, but employers felt that they could not employ him without front teeth. Luyanda became increasingly despondent. He seldom appeared to get joy out of the things that used to make him happy, including playing soccer. His motivation to look for work was steadily waning.

I had found a dentist in the private sector who agreed to work on Luyanda's teeth for free. I hoped that this would help to lift his spirits. But on a car journey from Khayelitsha to visit the dentist, Luyanda spoke of his other worries. He had been having problems with Andiswa. With his face turned away from me to hide his tears, Luyanda explained that Andiswa had been seeing other men. Hurt and ashamed, he understood why she would want to date someone with money. Luyanda did not want to leave Andiswa; he loved her and wished to stay with her, despite the fact that she had cheated on him. Luyanda's own father had died when he was young, and he spoke often about not having had a father figure in his life. He did not want the same for his daughter.

When his false tooth was fitted and the other tooth built up, Luyanda was happier than I had seen him in a long time. Over a year since he had lost his front teeth, Luyanda had become so accustomed to hiding his teeth that he took much convincing to expose his new smile.

Luyanda attempted to maintain and reinforce his identity as a young Xhosa man, but he also challenged some predominant understandings of hegemonic masculinity, while also illustrating how having a child as a teenager can represent a rational strategy to transition to adulthood.

For young couples like Luyanda and Andiswa, relationship stability and longevity was tested, partially achieved, or perceived to be bolstered through having a child. For Luyanda, becoming a father and demonstrating that he was in a stable, adult relationship acted as symbols of moving towards an accepted form of social adulthood, however tenuous that may have been.

Luyanda as a man, a father and an adult

Xhosa masculinity is informed by cultural practices, social relationships, material aspirations and religious beliefs (Mfecane 2016). These are drawn from a set of persistent ideals linked to the performance of dominant, hegemonic masculinity that inform what young men hope to achieve and aspire to in adulthood (Connell 2005).

Displays of strength, dominance and power are often regarded as synonymous with hegemonic masculinity, as are – in the context of poverty and uncertainty – more violent behaviours among men and boys from a young age (Bhana 2005). Luyanda's involvement in a youth gang offered him an avenue through which to prove his masculine strength, both to his peers and to the young women with whom he may have hoped to have sexual relationships. The ideal of male dominance over women, and the display of physical strength in relation to other men, may be performed through acts of violence and sexual violence, including in the context of young men's inability to meet the expectations associated with multiple sexual partners or capacity to provide for a woman or family. Young men's fear of losing or disappointing female partners may also lead them to attempt to prove their dominance through the use of force, in an attempt to mask their fears, doubts and vulnerabilities (Hunter 2005).

Luyanda was particularly concerned with his physical appearance. He wanted to be seen as muscular and strong, and he thought carefully about how he dressed to illustrate this. He worried about what his missing front tooth might communicate to others. Although he never expressed it explicitly, I sensed that his missing tooth symbolised his poverty – he was unable to pay for what was considered cosmetic dentistry. It also symbolised his exposure to a particular kind of violence associated with township life – bricks flying through the air in a gang fight are not uncommon.

But Luyanda's concern over his missing tooth was not only about the presentation of self; it was also closely linked to his attempts to find paying work to provide for his daughter. A persistent hegemonic masculine ideal is that men are financially independent and are able to provide for their girlfriends, wives and children (Bhana & Pattman 2011). The provision of material and financial resources to female sexual partners is a central aspect of initiating and maintaining sexual partnerships, as is discussed above (and also in case studies 2.5, 3.4 and 3.5). Giving a female partner gifts and paying for things (consumables, food, services) are seen as important in demonstrating love and affection, but also in proving the legitimacy of the relationship (Leclerc-Madlala 2009).

For most young men in townships, achieving complete financial independence is impossible (Bhana & Pattman 2011). Having a child often presents insurmountable costs for young parents, financially and in terms of the reproductive labour required to raise a child. As has been shown in case studies covering other townships, in Khayelitsha the overwhelming majority of households are multigenerational and headed by women (Posel & Devey 2006). Although residential fatherhood is uncommon, young fathers are beginning to play an important role in the lives of their children and their parents (Clark, Cotton et al. 2015; Swartz & Bhana 2009). This was true for Luyanda. The financial burden of caring for children was often spoken about in relation to the cost of nappies (diapers) – in excess of R200 (US$18) per pack – the equivalent for Luyanda of two full days of work, excluding the cost of transport to get to work or food to eat on those days. Like many young fathers, Luyanda was unable to achieve the ideal of the 'provider masculinity' to which he aspired (Bhana & Pattman 2011).

Many young people like Luyanda actively try to conceive as a way to build or test their relationships. Young people talked about wanting to 'create that bond' through having a child with a partner, to 'connect' the pair forever. Luyanda saw having a child with Andiswa as a way for him to check 'how things went' before asking her to marry him. Andiswa agreed. They were attempting to build, but also test, their existing relationship, and to show to each other their suitability for a long-term relationship because of their capacity to conceive.

Heterosexual sex is significant for hegemonic masculinity (Luyt 2012). The dominant image of African masculinity that is socially acceptable, even desirable, is to have multiple sexual partners (Delius & Glaser 2002; Mfecane 2008). Suzanne Leclerc-Madlala (2009) argues that African male sexuality is culturally scripted as 'unrestrainable'. Women should expect and endure their male partner's infidelity because men cannot be expected to go without sex when their partners are not available. Conversely, the dominant sexual script and social ideal of femininity is that women are chaste; if they are unfaithful, men should not stay in a partnership with them. This was inverted for Luyanda and Andiswa.

Andiswa's infidelity left Luyanda hurt and humiliated. Maintaining his relationship with Andiswa was one way for him to show that he was living up to an ideal he saw as linked to being a good father. Luyanda's own father had played no role in his life; he was determined that his daughter have a different experience. Luyanda therefore maintained his relationship with Andiswa out of his love for his daughter, and in an attempt to be seen by others as a good father.

Having a child was also an important avenue by which Luyanda could prove his virility and fertility to potential future partners. Luyanda once told me, 'If you don't have a photocopy [child], you need to get checked.' Other young men had a longer-term view in mind, and told their female partners that they wanted to have a child to prove that they could be 'good fathers', thus pointing to the future of their relationships and performances of masculinity.

Thus far, we have emphasised the role of families and households in biological reproduction – that is, pregnancy, birth and early infant care. The household is also the primary site of cultural reproduction, although family members who live separately may play a supplementary and supportive role. In this setting the physical and emotional care of infants and small children largely takes place: the support of their development, acquisition of skills, language, and ways of social interaction; and the values reflected by these. In addition, the household, not the family, is the site of daily reproduction, and the work involved in this. Such work takes place within a variety of dwellings – a basic RDP house, a larger privately owned suburban house, a townhouse, an inner-city apartment, or a shack. On a daily basis people need to meet personal-care needs, so they need to have access to bathing and toilet facilities, and to water to drink and with which to cook food and clean dishes, household surfaces and clothes. They also need fuel to cook and some source of power for lighting.

Some of these conditions can be met with little cash, but food is increasingly purchased and not grown, and people must often stretch limited budgets to ensure all householders are fed. People on very low and irregular incomes, whether or not in receipt of a state grant, have a particularly difficult time ensuring enough to eat; a 'good' diet or 'adequate' nutrition may be beyond their reach (D'Agostino et al. 2018; Rogan 2018; Zembe-Mkabile et al. 2018). In case study 4.3, which follows, Rebecca Hodes draws on data from research conducted in Johannesburg in 2017, using a mixed-method approach from economic anthropology (James 2014: 22) and inspired by earlier research on the interrelationship of consumption and identity-formation in South Africa (Hyslop 2005; Posel 2010). The research aimed to explore the small-scale, local-level purchasing practices of young South Africans. It was based within a broader study on the health of young South Africans, the Mzantsi Wakho study (Cluver et al. 2016; Hodes et al. 2018). The research combined discussion and interviews with a practical, participatory exercise: the 'grants shopping basket'. This exercise was conceptualised together with the study participants, and findings were analysed collaboratively. In the case study, Hodes describes how a couple dependent on a Child Support Grant for their infant's and their own needs made decisions about the purchase of food and other supermarket and baby products. She highlights how the young man in the couple was involved in and had a say in these decisions. Although during the exercise the young man and young woman in the couple made different choices, their strategies were remarkably similar: they stretched their budget by searching for items that were reduced or on special, and bought food that ensured their small child had a nutritious diet and so would be healthy.

Case study 4.3

The grants shopping basket

Rebecca Hodes

Precarity and ingenuity

I worked with a young couple – Joy (24) and Malusi (25). Both had been employed as researchers on the Mzantsi Wakho study,[1] but they had moved from the study's setting to another province when Joy became pregnant in 2015. For the birth of their daughter, Khomotso, they wanted to be nearer Joy's mother and sisters, trusted family members who could help with childcare. Joy's mother had survived a stroke in 2014, but her movement and speech were affected, and she had been unable to resume work. Previously, she had worked as a caterer and hawker – preparing meals at her home and selling them with other food at stands near to factories and businesses. While Joy's mother helped to care for Khomotso, she also required care from Joy, her sisters, and Malusi, particularly in the early months after her stroke as she slowly regained some movement and speech. Malusi's parents had both passed away in the late 1990s, and his closest relatives (a brother and sister) lived in different provinces. Arguments over family resources, including Malusi's requests for financial support from his sister, had strained their relationship, and he was no longer on good terms with his sister, his only sibling with a steady income.

Since leaving their jobs in the Eastern Cape, neither Joy nor Malusi had found regular employment. They sought work continuously and creatively, 'hustling' for wages as casual workers, including as shop assistants in a local mall, and in the businesses of their families and friends. But the costs of seeking work – including airtime for their cellphones, CV-printing, and travelling for interviews – were often prohibitive. As Joy explained: 'I've written letters of motivation. I've sent forms. But if I don't have an income at all, it costs me … I don't have a safety net, so I am falling on this pointy stuff … With all my heart, I just want to work. I need to work.'

Joy's mother's house was in Hammanskraal, about 50 kilometres from Pretoria, where Joy had grown up. Her mother shared the house with Joy's two younger sisters. Owing to space constraints in the house, Joy, Malusi and their one-year-old daughter moved into a rented room in Hammanskraal. Through an illegal connection, Joy and Malusi had access to electricity, but their rental costs were high, using most of their income. When we met, they had not yet been able to buy basic furnishings for their room, including a fridge or a bed. For the previous three months or so, they had slept on cardboard and blankets, and had subsisted mostly on dry goods (samp, rice and beans) that could be stored without cooling. They relied on limited and haphazard financial support from relatives, but the Child Support Grant (CSG) was their principal, recurrent source of household income. They spent it to feed and look after Khomotso, and to subsist themselves.

The 'grants shopping basket' exercise that formed part of the research on which this case study is based was conducted at a large supermarket in Johannesburg. The exercise had three components. First, Joy and Malusi each filled a shopping basket with products that they would ordinarily purchase with the grant, not exceeding the total of R374. They were asked to do the exercise individually, and to avoid discussing or comparing their baskets' contents while passing each other in the aisles. Second, items purchased (using an audited research fund for participatory research on social support) were divided into packets indicating who had chosen them. We carried them to a quiet venue, where we unpacked and discussed them. Third, through negotiation and compromise, Joy and Malusi consolidated their purchases, deciding which products to keep and which to remove. The result was a selection of items that represented their mutually construed needs and decisions for household provision. Figure 4.1 shows the items Joy and Malusi individually chose. Figure 4.2 shows the selection of items after they consolidated their purchases.

Two findings based on this exercise are described below. First, Joy and Malusi spent most of the grant on food and cleaning products for their baby. Their principal objective was to provide for Khomotso's nutrition and sanitation, while ensuring their own subsistence. Second, Joy and Malusi used a range of tactics to 'stretch' the grant: seeking out bargains and specials; purchasing 'no name' generic products; and choosing food items, cleaning products and toiletries of use to all.

Figure 4.1 *Grants shopping basket: Individually chosen items*

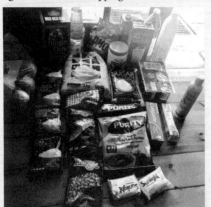 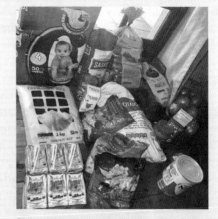

Malusi	Joy
Apples R12.99	Cuddlers nappies R109.99
Carrots (small) R8.99	No name rice 2 kg pack R15.99
Jungle Oats R23.99	Juice pack long life – apple R3.99
Noodles (four packs): R3.99 × 4 = R15.96	Juice pack long life – pineapple R9.99
No name vinegar R7.99	Sasko cake flour R19.99
No name rice R37.78	Lucky Star pilchards R15.99
No name tea R8.99 (image not shown in the photograph)	Panado strawberry syrup R33.99
Red speckled sugar beans (two bags): R13.99 × 2 = R27.98	Three packets macaroni on special at 3 for R14.99
Omo washing powder R18.99	Potatoes R35.00
Aqueous cream R29.99	Carrots (bulk) R21.00
No name brown sugar R16.99	Tomatoes R21.00
Purity baby's porridge (two bags): R14.99 × 2 = R29.98	Gem squash R15.99
Sunlight soap (two bars): R5.49 × 2 = R10.98	Onions R23.00
No name brand full cream milk long life (2 litres) R11.99 × 2 = R23.98	Peanut butter R24.99
Nutriday yoghurt R13.79	Polony R4.69
Colgate toothpaste R9.99	Nido formula milk R65.99
Milk teeth children's toothpaste R10.00	Ashton and Parsons infants' powders R27.99
No name cooking oil R16.99	
No name bleach R7.99	
Hair oil/moisturiser R23.99	
Total R358.33 (Underspent by R15.67)	**Total R443.57** (Overspent by R69.57)

Figure 4.2 *Grants shopping basket: Combined selection, Joy and Malusi*

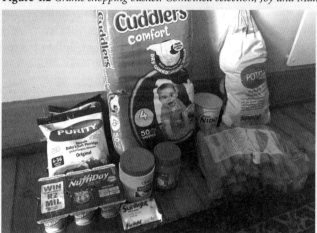

Joy and Malusi

Cuddlers nappies R109.99
Purity baby's porridge (2 bags): R14.99 x 2 = R29.98
Nutriday yoghurt R13.79
Bar Sunlight soap R5.49
Aqueous cream R29.99
Peanut butter R24.99
Nido formula milk R65.99
Carrots (bulk) R21.00
Potatoes R35.00
TOTAL R336.22   (Underspent by R37.78)

'The first priority is the best, healthy food'

Joy and Malusi both described their main objective as securing and advancing the health and nutrition of their child. They chose the best foods available and affordable, considering ingredients lists and avoiding unhealthy chemicals to protect and advance their daughter's health. In choosing sorghum porridge and beans, Malusi explained:

> The ingredients here, they are better than any porridge that you will get.
> There are other porridges … but those fancy ones tend to have too much
> of banana flavours and colourants and every stuff … The first priority is
> the best, healthy food for the child, is that porridge. That's why I got this.
> And the beans … There's a soup that comes from it that you cook it with,
> the broth, and that's what we feed our children because it has nutritional
> benefit for them.

Joy selected a range of fresh fruits and vegetables to provide 'seven colours' of fresh produce – inspired by the maxim that fresh foods of various colours ensure a broad nutritional spectrum. 'She needs butternut, she needs carrots, she needs potato,' Joy explained. Yoghurt was selected for its calcium content, and beans for their protein (as a substitute for meat, which was expensive to buy and difficult to keep without refrigeration).

Besides food, sanitation products – nappies, soap and cream – were the main purchases. Malusi chose toothpaste for infants and young children, and hair-conditioning oil; Joy chose a paracetamol-containing syrup and baby powders to soothe teething pains and fevers. Again, the health and wellbeing of their child were foremost, but Khomotso's appearance and presentability, in the gaze of others, was also important. The creams and hair lotions would ensure that Khomotso looked healthy and well-provided for, as Malusi explained: 'I don't want my child to look like that maybe in front of other people. But you know what Joy will be worried about? She will be so worried that, eish, Khomotso's hair is dry, and I don't like it when she goes out like this.'

Khomotso's appearance reflected Joy's and Malusi's aspiration to appear successful, despite their economic realities and living circumstances. Khomotso's visible wellbeing and health, as reflected in public, indicated this positive achievement, contrasting with their socioeconomic constraints, unemployment, and dependence upon state support.

> Joy: For me, my biggest concern, I feel like your child sometimes, when you walk at the mall, is a reflection of your status. People use children as status. I'm always concerned that, I want people when they look at Khomotso, to not feel sorry for her, that she symbolises the state that I'm in in my life, that I'm still trying to pick up my life, or how struggling I am. So I always want to cover that, to do what's best for her. When I look at her, I always want her to have Nido, because when I look at Nido I feel like, as much as if I cannot have veggies for the whole week, and she has this, her body is still getting something.

> Malusi: She's getting a nutritional thing, *ja*.

> Joy: Because kids can show poverty at the best level. Their eyes turn red, their skin just cracks. They are just able to show that you are poor if you don't work and cover that up. Me and Malusi, we can live without for a week without cream, without body cream.

> Malusi: *Ja*.

> Joy: But put Khomotso for a week without a body cream, it's horrible. It's scary for a parent to see a child like this.

Malusi: One thing that Joy said is that, 'You know, people from school they always knew me as this bright person, and they always–'

Joy: 'Expected the best–'

Malusi: Expected that thing that maybe they will see me driving a car one day. So now when they see me with a child, they must at least see my child as best. They may not see me as best, but they must at least see my child as best, because my child is a representative of what I have, of everything that I would be.

'I always like the specials'

In planning grocery lists and deciding where to shop, Malusi and Joy searched for bargains and specials. They scanned the advertising sections of newspapers, looking for promotions. During the 'grants shopping basket' exercise, they selected items that were on special. They also chose not to buy a larger quantity of particular staples – including maize meal – on the basis that this was less expensive at their local supermarket and also (they knew from experience) of a better quality. Reviewing Joy's purchases, Malusi recounted, 'The other thing that I know always makes [Joy] to buy this thing, from all these options, is the specials … Because she can buy even more.' Joy agreed, 'I always like the specials.'

Both Joy and Malusi explained their selection of certain products according to discounts, and recalled the exact costs of these discounted items, mostly without reference to the till slip. Describing his product selection, Malusi priced each from memory, rounding off costs to ensure that he did not go over budget, and recollecting which items he had chosen because they were on special. The interview transcript captures this scrutiny:

This one was also on special. This was R9.99, R10, so it's R70. I still remember, this was R14.99, R15. So, it's 70 rands, it's 85. Then so there's R15 left, then you can just sort it out all, and say it's R100. Fine. *Ja*, it's R20, *ja*, it's R100. Then, you go to the milk, it was R10.99. This aqueous is R29.99, it's expensive, because there's R5.00 difference at this shop. This is R41 [R20 and R21 for carrots and tomatoes], it's R41 plus R23 [Jungle Oats], it's R64, right? R64 plus R5, then its R69 [realises he's made a mistake], yoh, sorry, it's R10, so it's R64, R64. Four, 8, 12, 16, it's R74. R74 plus R8.99 [carrots], then this one is R4.00 [long life still apple], so it's R104; 104 rands, then this one is cheap, it's R8, it's R104 plus 8, 4 plus 8 is 12.

Joy made similar calculations:

> I know about every one, how much each costs. I did my calculations right. [Pointing to items and identifying their cost.] This is R33, this is R27, R9, R9, R10, R18, R15. R15. This is a special [pointing to a packet of macaroni], 3 of them for R15.

Both Joy and Malusi described how buying discounted items helped to extend their budgets. But, this potential offsetting of costs had to be weighed against other considerations, including the product's shelf-life (often discounted items were nearing expiry date), time and energy required for preparation (pasta, for instance, required more time to prepare than instant porridge), and whether the items on promotion were essential, or whether their reduced price had elevated their desirability and seeming utility.

The CSG was conceived of as a means of supplementing household incomes and directing funds to the education and wellbeing of children. But, in the context of soaring unemployment and the absence of other income sources, it is the principal source of revenue for millions of households. It also affects the caring practices and is the subject of intense public debate. Despite evidence which shows the contrary, in popular discourse widespread allegations abound about people who abuse the CSG. In such allegations misspending is attributed to both a lack (of parsimony, parental responsibility and financial literacy) and a profusion (of the desire for luxurious, superfluous or dangerous consumer products – such as beauty products or alcohol). As I illustrate here, financial and material acuity undergirds the grant's expenditure. By examining a couple's grants shopping basket, analysing its contents, and studying the processes through which items are selected, I have demonstrated how one young family enacts the 'calculus of care', according to which they must balance the necessity of their household's subsistence with the objective of providing for their child.

South Africa is unique in specifying protection in the Bill of Rights (Chapter 2 of the Constitution) from discrimination on the basis of sex, gender and sexual orientation. Yet this does not prevent homophobia, sexism, or xenophobic or other standpoints that are contrary to the spirit and intent of the Constitution, and it does not necessarily lead men to rethink their roles and relationships to others.

In the following case study (4.4), Mzikazi Nduna and Welmari Bouwer draw on research with young Afrikaner men, rarely a subject of research in South Africa. The research was conducted in a lower-middle-class area of Pretoria West, approximately 50 kilometres outside Pretoria. Ten young Afrikaner men, aged from 15 to 18 years, who (to their knowledge) were not yet fathers, participated in the study. White Afrikaans-speaking South Africans make up 4 per cent of the total population, with historical links to Afrikaner nationalism and its oppression of other South Africans prior to and under apartheid. This is also a community that, with shifts from small-scale to commercial farming, is relatively poor. Orthodox Christianity feeds conservatism, and conventional views about reproduction, family structure (Botha 2017), fatherhood and masculinity. For men who grew up living without a father, or whose relationship with their fathers was troubled, these ideals again reflect local ideologies, and not lived experience.

Case study 4.4

On being a father

Mzikazi Nduna and Welmari Bouwer

Marriage is considered an important step towards family formation by the heterosexual Afrikaner community (Macleod & Morison 2015). Families are characterised by relatively strict gender roles in domestic life, with men seen as the 'head of the household' and women playing strongly supportive roles. In general, fathering in Afrikaans households reflects a hypermasculine role. The ideal man is physically tough and brave, able to provide materially for the family and to fulfil non-nurturing roles, including that of spiritual leader (Koenig-Visagie & Van Eeden 2013). However, increasing demands on workforce participants to work longer hours and travel from home has led to the increased absence of men in families (Viljoen 2011). While the role of primary breadwinner remains dominant, it is not sustainable for all white Afrikaans men, due to changes in economic policies and employment prospects (Koenig-Visagie & Van Eeden 2013). In addition, separation, divorce, single parenthood and death all shape the structure of households.

Of the 10 young men who participated in the study, 8 lived with their biological mother, and either had a stepfather or received assistance from their maternal grandmother. These different configurations occurred for various reasons. Divorce was one, despite the disapproval of the Afrikaans community, reflecting Christian ideology regarding the sanctity of marriage (Macleod & Morison 2015). One participant, Kobus, said:

> Your parents just think, okay no, it's cool, we divorce now, we are now getting out of the relationship, it is okay. But they do not know what they do to the children. It is a scar for life actually, if I think about it now. It's literally, it touches you … It affects you very much.

A second reason was the death of the father, which resulted in financial hardship, as another participant, Daan, described: 'It is tough now because now we – The circumstances are very difficult and … yeah. It was hard for me. Now we are struggling a lot.' Similar adversities emerged for young men because of substance use by parents. In cases such as Albert's, substance use coexisted with domestic violence, leading him to want to escape his living arrangements.

In households where the father was entirely absent, participants lamented the lack of consistent financial and physical support: 'I don't know, my father, it's as if he wasn't interested anymore. He only pays R650 alimony a month. It's not actually a lot. That's enough to get me to school and back' (Nico). In other cases, fathers' absence was not constant, and in certain instances, father and son reconnected when the father moved closer, as Albert explained: 'He lives just so around the bend from us. Now I see him every weekend. Instead of talking on a phone, I talk to him face to face.' Dirk's situation was similar: 'Now I go to him in the afternoons. He's a lot better than my stepdad. He doesn't shout at me.'

Research from a study of African men who grew up without their fathers suggests that significant others fill the void created by an absent father (Clowes et al. 2013; Langa 2010). However, these findings, and research with other Afrikaans-speaking communities, suggest the significance of gendered child rearing requiring a competent father (however defined) for a son (Macleod & Morison 2015). In this context, women were not seen as capable of fulfilling the paternal role, and participants here, as elsewhere (Vilanculos & Nduna 2017), believed in stereotypical gender roles. Sons needed fathers 'to teach them all the things about life. I don't think a father can teach a lot of things to their daughters' (Jan).

White Afrikaans male participants naturalised the connection of sex (male), character (masculine), and role (fatherhood), and the absent biological father was constructed as a deficit: 'It is just important for me to have a dad because a dad is the man in a house. If your dad is not there, then what do you do?' (Albert); 'It's been tough living without a father. The way I am these days is very different compared to what I used to be … I used to have that manly figure there, my father' (Daan); 'I, to be honest, I think my – I think your dad, children who grow up without a dad have a much harder, harder life than normal children' (Kobus).

The role of the father is expected to be filled by others (Davies & Eagle 2013), and participants had other adult males: 'It's basically family like my uncle. He is very close to us and yeah, he helps us a lot. And yes, and, and when, when I greet him then he gives me a hug. It feels to me as if he is a father' (Daan); 'I have many uncles that I like … that I would have liked to be my dad' (Willem).

Pieter said,

> Eh, my stepdad … my mother met him around when I think I was in Grade two. So, I have known him for about 15 years or something now. Ah yeah I sort of do like him, he's actually sort of a good dad. He has, he takes care of me and all those things.

Participants defined a 'social father' as a man who provided them with emotional and sometimes financial support. In one instance, the role of the social father was taken up by an older brother. Kobus described the responsibilities placed on him, and how he was happy to help take care of his younger brother. He did not, however, wish to be regarded as a father figure.

Stepfathers may ease the financial and childcare burden placed on a single-mother household, although the entry of the 'other' – the mother's new partner – was not always easy. Participants monitored and scrutinised their stepfather's behaviour. At times a stepfather was regarded as inconsequential, but at other times he was abusive, violent towards his partner, and subjected her family to abuse and financial struggles. Daan hoped that his mother would not date whilst he was still at home, to avoid tension. Willem described the unpredictable behaviour of his stepfather:

> He broke more of my things than what he bought for me. Like … it was my birthday, then I got an Xbox or something just for a couple of weeks. Then we had to sell it for money. Then [he] had a job, just worked a few weeks, and then he doesn't like the job and then he sits at the house.

Growing up with an absent father

Even for participants who did grow up without their biological fathers, the influence of the single mother was not powerful enough to unsettle ideas of 'doing gender'. The gendered scripts and separation of breadwinner from caretaker roles were evident in young men's views of fatherhood and fathering. Albert (15) and Daan (17) both believed that it was the man's duty to perform manual labour and to ensure the house was safe: 'Uh, the man in the house must be there to, to protect you. So, if someone breaks in, then there is an adult man who can protect you' (Albert); 'And I think if you have a father and he lives there, he should make sure that the house is safe and he should do all the basic things like cutting the grass, the garden and things like that' (Daan).

In participants' minds, the role of providing a safe and secure environment would not transfer to a woman; protection was a man's duty (see also Macleod & Morison 2015). This contrasted with the domestic roles that they expected woman to undertake. However, when asked whose responsibility it was to take care of the child, Nico (18) and Pieter (18), whose mothers worked, encouraged greater involvement by men: 'The mom and the dad. It is both genders or from both. It has to come from both sides, to yeah become closer to each other' (Nico); 'I think my stepdad and my mom, they say luckily, but everyone just has to help where they can' (Pieter).

Almost all participants firmly stated that they loved their mothers, and commented on the amount of work they did for their family. Participants also voiced their desire to protect their mothers from perceived harm, as a manly duty and a selfless obligation. Albert described his preventative measures: 'No, he [stepfather] would not hit her. I will do something to him. Yes. I love my mom a lot. That's why if she works night shift then I don't sleep out. I sleep at the house.'

Fatherhood in the future

Although our participants grew up without their biological fathers, they did not think about fatherhood as a choice. Fatherhood was constructed as normative, an inevitable outcome and the missing puzzle-piece of a marriage. This finding resonates with the assumptions of the heteronormative matrix and the 'marriage–procreation bond' (Macleod & Morison 2015). While participants considered that staying married was optional in the case of discord, they saw children as a reason to stay, even if they were unhappy: 'Say now I'm one day married. And I'm not content with the relationship that I have. Then I will make sure to stay in that relationship, until my children are big enough to care for themselves, like if … they are already 18' (Kobus).

A sporting life

Whilst experiences with an absent father are familiar in research on absent fathers in South Africa, what distinguishes this group was the importance of rugby in South African Afrikaans culture. Rugby events are described as offering familial bonding experiences and were seen to be an important part of Afrikaans culture. Young men had fond memories of times when their biological father was present: 'In the afternoons when I got home from school, then we played rugby outside on the grass' (Daan). When the father was absent, this was deeply felt: 'Just that he should have been there. Like when I was growing up. Like, for example, my first rugby game, my cricket game. And when I broke my collar bone' (Jan). For some participants, the absence of their father at sporting events influenced the importance they placed on their presence for their own future children. They suggested: 'If I have a child I would really like to be a father who will stand by him through everything, sport— all sorts of sport' (Hendrik); 'I would really like to be involved, if you have a sport opportunity. I would actually want to be there for him or for her' (Pieter).

Whilst father absence is not unusual – in any setting or society – the meanings and implications for affected children are created, co-created, and responded to in context. No matter what the child's current relationship with their biological father was, participants always made a clear distinction between a biological father and other 'father figures' such as a stepfather, uncle or grandfather. Despite displaying a vested interest in their lives, social fathers were not considered to be a substitute for the biological father. Further, young men drew attention to the difficulties when a man's presence was inconsistent. This suggests the importance of support to households where family composition is disrupted or fluid.

Case studies 4.1 to 4.4 focus on fatherhood and parenting, but the role of men in households and with family members extends beyond this. In case study 4.5, we turn to self-care, and to how men think about their physical and social bodies.

By 2017, the life expectancy of men and women had increased dramatically as a result of antiretroviral therapy (ART), but even so, there was a marked difference by sex. In 2017, life expectancy at birth for men was estimated at 61.5 years, and for women at 67.7 years (Stats SA 2019).

Despite the apparent better outcomes for women, other health indicators identified in the most recent census illustrate the influences of gender on health. For instance, women are more likely to report hunger, because of the greater levels of poverty of female-headed households. According to government statistics, women are more likely than men to have chronic health problems, but they are also more likely to contract acute illnesses and to sustain more injuries. They more often provide care to children and grandchildren, and are the primary caregivers of ageing spouses, parents, parents-in-law, and adult children unable to live independently. The work of care also includes self-care – including diet, exercise, and whether one seeks care from a formal provider if need be. But, as the following case study illustrates, this does not imply passivity. The two men introduced in case study 4.5 – both with limited income – explain their own care practices in relation to everyday diet, incidental exercise, personal practices and their understandings of vulnerability. In this respect, their ambivalence to women, and the perceived threat of female sexuality to men's bodies and health, is laid bare. The case study draws on ethnographic research conducted by Edmond Madhuha in 2016–2017 in the small town of Modimolle, Limpopo Province.

Case study 4.5

Responsible masculinity

Edmond Madhuha and Lorena Núñez Carrasco

This case study draws on the experiences of two men – Halimani and Tumelo, who live in two very different areas of Modimolle, Limpopo Province (Madhuha 2017) – to explore how their working-class position impacts their health and how their notions of health and wellbeing relate to gender relations. At the centre of their practices to stay healthy, *maikarabelo* (responsible masculinity) emerges as a driving force in men's health practices. Informed by cultural notions about gender and sexuality, *maikarabelo* also prescribes when sexual encounters might be harmful, by specifying the conditions under which a sexual partner might be considered polluting and dangerous.

Halimani is 47 years old and has lived in Modimolle all his life; he is divorced and, at the time of the research, had a new partner. They have been living together for 18 months and are still considering a long-term commitment. They have a young boy. They live in a government-built (RDP) house. Although there are no paved roads where Halimani lives, the services offer better conditions for residents' health compared to the informal settlement where Tumelo lives, which lacks basic services. Halimani is a cash-in-transit security officer, and his job is to handle cash from different companies operating in Modimolle. His day at work starts at 7 a.m. when he is dropped off by a company car, and ends at 6 p.m. when he walks for one hour back home. Every day he collects money from four different companies and takes this to the bank, and waits until the bank tellers have finalised reconciling the cash. He is constantly on the move. He needs to be very alert and in control, always armed with a gun and clad in a bulletproof vest. The pace of work and the risk of handling cash makes Halimani's job stressful; he is always on his feet. He describes his work:

> Starting at 10 a.m. until 3 p.m., I would be on my feet with no time to sit down. From 10 to 3, I will be on my feet and not in the car, but I will be in the bank where I will be cashing in the money, counting it to make sure it tallies.

Some companies request he brings change from the bank – in most cases coins – so he has to carry heavy boxes of coins. This makes his work physically very demanding. The routine is the same throughout the week. Halimani returns home tired at around 7 p.m. to the care of his partner, who prepares the evening meal. On Saturdays, when he doesn't work, he wakes up around 5 a.m., and jogs until 7 a.m.:

> I exercise and when I come back, before taking a bath, I get into my garden and take care of my vegetables since it [his garden] also needs attention like a human being for it to survive. Just as a human being bathes, the garden also needs attention, so I water the vegetables and use a garden fork to loosen the soil for aeration. After finishing I take my bath and maybe around two in the afternoon I start to drink beer. On a day, I smoke about three to four cigarettes. I am a person who loves exercising so that I become healthy in my body. I don't just sit.

In his small yard, Halimani has planted spinach and potatoes, an important contribution to the food security of the household. Halimani is conscious about his health. He says, 'I like vegetables too much. I don't like to eat meat that much.' He expands:

> Health needs you to take care of yourself, not just to sit and think that it's nothing. Training makes you healthy; the food you eat makes you healthy in your body. So, if you eat without exercising you become overweight and you can even fail to walk. You don't live well in the end. If you don't exercise and you are eating fatty foods, it makes you to become obese such that you fail even to walk for three kilometres. I think that if you eat healthy foods like vegetables and meat and you exercise, you become healthy.

Tumelo lives in a shack in an informal settlement without basic sanitation. Public taps were placed strategically in the informal settlement, but became dry during a drought. Residents have dug underground wells for water for domestic use. Makeshift pit toilets have been dug in the same area; when full, they are simply closed off and new pit toilets are made. Some of the men claim that they experience stomach pains and need to attend the local clinic, but Tumelo insists the well water is safe:

> I think the water is safe because we cover the opening with some materials
> so that nothing can fall into the well. Since we started having the water,
> we have never complained about it. If the water was not safe, by now we
> would have closed these wells and there were supposed to be complaints
> of stomach pains and stuff but there is nothing like that since these wells
> have started two years ago [i.e. since 2015].

Tumelo is 31 years old and he lives with his partner and child. He has worked for the last seven years at a brick-making company, some 20 kilometres outside Modimolle town. He wakes up at 5 a.m. and prepares his lunch box for work. He works from 7 a.m. until 4.30 p.m., and he gets home around 5 p.m.. The company provides transport to and from work. His work involves packing bricks, and he is paid at a piece rate with daily targets expected to be met. In the production chain, Tumelo packs the bricks to be burned in a furnace: 'The work is tough, and it is heavy. It calls for one's endurance; if you are not able to persevere you cannot make it.' His workplace is full of dust from the bricks. Tumelo has his own ways to protect himself from dust particles both from the burning bricks and from general dust:

> You are supposed to drink milk, in actual fact you are not supposed to
> take one week without drinking Ultra Mel [long-life milk, able to be used
> unopened without refrigeration] so that the milk can unblock the dust
> fumes from your lungs so that you can breathe properly, otherwise the
> dust will make you sick by causing tuberculosis.

Tumelo is concerned about his future because of the hard conditions of his job. He considered finding a more skilled job, like becoming an excavator operator. However, this would require vocational college training. He hopes to continue his role as breadwinner, and this drives him to pursue new opportunities for his life. As he puts it, the reason to look for new job opportunities is 'so that I can be able to feed my children, you see.' Even though with the money he gets he can afford to take care of his family, his work has a negative effect on his health: 'Remember when you perspire you lose weight and as a human being you are not supposed to lose weight too much.' Referring to the kind of food he eats at home, Tumelo says:

> In most cases I like to eat *pap* [porridge] and vegetables, especially spinach.
> I am not able to spend three or four days without eating spinach. A lot of
> people around here have small gardens and sometimes I get it from them.
> I like vegetables because they help your body system. The soldiers of the
> body are strengthened so that they are able to function properly.

Tumelo's reasoning for eating porridge is that it 'lasts longer in his body' and gives him the necessary energy for physical work. Tumelo also acknowledges the role his wife plays – she cooks and provides him with water to bathe. In turn, he says, 'At the end of the month I am able to do what my family wants,' by providing for them. He acknowledges his wife is always by his side when he is not feeling well: 'She also feels the pain when I am sick.' Tumelo also takes leave from work to take care of his wife if she is not feeling well.

When he is off work, Tumelo likes to take care of his garden. He sometimes enjoys taking a walk to town, a distance of about 3.5 kilometres. Yet, due to his demanding work, Tumelo admits he sometimes just wants to rest when not working. To keep healthy, he uses 'Stameta [a detoxifying ingredient sold over the counter] just to clean my blood'. Stameta helps him to clean 'some dirt in the body and where the blood is not flowing properly, it [Stameta] opens up the valves of the body.' His body feels relieved after using this enema.

In the context of limited opportunities, these men draw from a pool of resources to look after their health and wellbeing: diet, physical exercise, and enemas.

Maikarabelo

Halimani's understanding of what it means to be a man is, 'If we say there is a man we mean he has *maikarabelo*' – this means a man is defined by the weight of responsibility he carries. Halimani adds, 'For example, he has a family, a home that is his; he takes full responsibility over the people under his household. That's what we can call a man.' *Maikarabelo*, in Sepedi, is responsible masculinity. Halimani emphasises that *maikarabelo* distinguishes a man from a boy:

> A person without responsibility, we cannot call him a man. We say he is
> still a boy because he does not support and he does not have a wife or
> children. How can we call such a person a man because to be a man you
> must have a family, children and a home? If you don't have those things we
> will still call you a boy since you still live under the roof of your parents.
> He doesn't have responsibility; there are no people that look for something
> from him. He is still interested in the pleasures of this world and he
> doesn't have responsibility. We cannot call him a man but he will continue
> to be a boy. But he who has *maikarabelo*, maybe he has children, a house
> and a wife – we can't call him a boy; we will say he is a man because he has
> reproduced himself on earth. He has children, a wife and a house and he
> has responsibility. He has other people that live because of him and that is
> why we say he is a man. He is the head of the family.

Most working-class men interviewed in the research subscribed to this notion. A man is defined by the responsibilities he carries on behalf of his household, as Tumelo explained:

> To say there is a man; people simply look at where you are living, how you treat the woman you are living with, whether you are able to provide for her and whether you are able to build a family. If you are a man, you are supposed to have a family and that means you are supposed to have a wife. You have to marry that wife. Everything that happens in the family is your responsibility. If you are a man you are supposed to have a family, have a wife and have children and marry. In the end, you must ensure children are well provided for.

Responsible masculinity revolves around a man's position to establish an independent family, a homestead or *umuzi* (Hunter 2005: 211) and assume household headship. If a man is not working, Halimani insists,

> Ja, he is still a man because yes, he was working but was retrenched, for example, those people are still his to take care of. He still takes care of them; it doesn't mean that now because he is not working, those people must reject him. No, because they are still living with him, he has a family and the home is still his to take care of. He is still a man. That cannot change.

Responsible masculinity is encapsulated by a man having the means to earn an income and to be able to lead, provide and care for his family. It is also anchored in how men take care of their health. In the face of flexible living arrangements resulting in high rates of cohabitation in informal settlements (Hunter 2005), and the acceptability of men's multiple sexual relations, working-class men express their fears around the pollution of the female body.

Risky gender relations and bodily pollution

Among all men interviewed, building one's own home was a major theme in the construction of masculinity and a mark of *maikarabelo*. Against this yardstick, the majority of men felt that it was acceptable for men to have other sexual relations (see Hunter 2005 on *isoka* masculinity), provided this was done in a responsible manner, and did not involve a polluted and dangerous woman – a pregnant woman (when he was not responsible for the pregnancy), a widow who had not yet been ceremonially cleansed, a woman who had recently aborted, or a woman who was menstruating. These men maintained that having sex with women in any of these circumstances could cause harm and was potentially fatal. Halimani pointed out:

> Yes, [this is] serious … have you not ever seen some men with swollen manhood by merely looking at them? It [the penis] will be swollen and it becomes watery when you have had sex with a widow. If you sleep with a woman who has aborted, you will be lucky to survive. Both cases

are similar, they work through the blood. It makes your blood not to be normal. It means that when your blood is not normal, blood works hand in hand with the heart. Now if the heart beats, your blood will be faster than the heart beat and what will happen? Blood is pumped by the heart for it to circulate in the body, now if the blood is now moving faster it means you are in danger. Having sex with a woman who has aborted will kill you. That one is dangerous … you sleep with her today and tomorrow, as that woman will leave your house you will remain in real danger. Your whole body will be in pain.

Halimani continued:

The thing is that woman is just dangerous [one who has had a recent abortion]. The funny part is that herself, she will be able to live, but you as a man who has slept with her will take her blood into your body and your health will deteriorate faster. In her case she will live a normal life but for you as a man you will not be able to live past a week. If you live with that secret and [do] not seek help, you will not be able to live past a month. It will be showing in your body that you are sick. That thing will eat and finish you off, it destroys your blood. If you were light in complexion for example, you will become darker because your blood is now dirty. That disease eats up your blood and destroys the soldiers of your body; it exhausts your strength, that's why it is even able to kill you.

Similarly, Tumelo spoke of how he narrowly survived from sleeping with a woman who was ritually unclean from a recent abortion. He had recently visited the hospital and, while initially reserved, he opened up and elaborated:

The problem was [hesitantly] … actually it was because of this issue with women. It is because I once slept with a lady who had terminated pregnancy, you see. So, it caused me a big problem such that I had to visit the hospital so that I could get help. That is the problem that I once faced. I was admitted at the hospital for a week and was given treatment.

Tumelo had consulted a traditional doctor about his condition:

I had slept with a woman who had aborted but she hid her condition from me, you see. The traditional healer performed the rituals and he told me that the woman I had sex with had aborted and that I had slept with her before she was cleansed. As a result, I took over the dirt from her and that was the cause of my sickness. I confronted the woman and asked her why she did not disclose to me that she had terminated pregnancy. It was then that she confessed and asked for forgiveness from me. I even took the traditional herbs prescribed by the traditional doctor. However, the treatment didn't really help me that much. It only temporarily helped me and in the end I realised I had to visit the hospital where I managed to get cured and now I am fine.

Tumelo went to hospital, where he was diagnosed with tuberculosis, but he is certain that his sickness derived from the sexual encounter.

We have described how men carve a particular kind of 'responsible' masculinity called *maikarabelo* in the context of limited opportunities. *Maikarabelo* is at the centre of how men define themselves as providers to their households and as household heads, and how they manage their own health and wellbeing through diet, physical activities, enema use and the use of both biomedicine and traditional healing within a plural healthcare system. Men's sexuality and concurrent sexual relations stretch this responsible masculinity. Responsible masculinity becomes a terrain of contestations and contradictions when men become entangled with 'polluted' women, risking possible death. The premise of responsible masculinity is embodied by these men in such sexual encounters, when women are seen as having the ultimate power to damage men.

Over the past two decades, there has been growing research in South Africa and globally on intimate-partner violence and gender-based violence, dominating other research on men and masculinity (Lundgren & Amin 2015; McCloskey 2016). In South Africa, population-based studies indicate that nearly a quarter of women have experienced physical and sexual violence from a partner by the age of 20, and up to 60 per cent experienced them over a lifetime, with long-term physical, social and mental health effects (Dartnall & Jewkes 2013; Selin et al. 2019). Men's violence against women has been contextualised against poverty, unemployment and social exclusion, with women – both intimate partners and others – on the receiving end of men's frustration at living in continued extreme inequality. But at the same time, the 'performance' of masculinity – including men's attitudes and behaviours such as aggression, dominance and ideas of sexual entitlement – is associated with men's violence to assert power and control (Gibbs et al. 2018).

In the following case study (4.6), Ruari-Santiago McBride and Mzwakhe Khumalo describe an intervention that was designed to transform gender relations and social norms. The setting is the township of Narrow Ridge (pseudonym) in urban Johannesburg, which developed differently from the older townships of Soweto or Khayelitsha, where previous case studies in this book have been based. The study was conducted from 2014 to 2016 and involved extended community engagement. In this setting, people live in extreme overcrowding, with substandard housing, a lack of basic amenities and infrastructure, and a lack of employment – a combination of conditions associated with men's violence, but not an excuse for it. The intervention is one of several involving NGOs (non-governmental organisations) across the country, working with men to question the norms that facilitate and enable violence. But, as the case study's authors argue, the structural contexts in which violence is most prevalent highlight the need also for sustained intersectoral engagement and political will to change.

Case study 4.6

Hitting out

Ruari-Santiago McBride and Mzwakhe Khumalo

Narrow Ridge (pseudonym) is a township located on the periphery of Johannesburg. It was established in 1994 when a community, which had occupied nearby farmland, was relocated there by the government. It grew as more people were resettled there from neighbouring townships. At the same time, white middle- and upper-class people were increasingly migrating from Johannesburg's city centre to suburban 'gated communities'. This pushed the city limits towards Narrow Ridge, which serendipitously found itself within commutable distance from some of Johannesburg's wealthiest communities and largest shopping malls. Narrow Ridge's strategic location made the township an attractive proposal for people searching out economic opportunities. The speed at which people came to Narrow Ridge outpaced public investment, and the area became densely populated. This resulted in high levels of deprivation in terms of income, employment, education, health and living environment.

The ad hoc development of Narrow Ridge led it to become a patchwork of 13 'extensions', with varied formality and accessibility to services. Some extensions include tarmac roads; street lighting; waste-disposal services; and brick houses with electricity, water and sanitation, built either as RDP houses or using private finance. Other extensions are highly informal, with narrow dirt roads; no public lighting, sewage or waste disposal services; and sheet-metal houses that are served by communal taps and toilets. A few extensions mix formal and informal housing.

Narrow Ridge has two public health clinics, a police station, a library, a skills-development and youth centre, and a park. Although the physical and social infrastructure is greater than what is available in many townships, on the whole Narrow Ridge lacks the social services, cultural opportunities and recreational facilities expected of an urban community of its size, especially when compared to nearby gated communities with smaller populations. Furthermore, the limited services available in Narrow Ridge are not equally accessible to all residents, since emergency-response services – such as police and ambulances – do not access informal areas out of fear and due to the narrowness of the roads.

Narrow Ridge has a notorious reputation for violence, particularly against women. Exceptionally high numbers of men report that they have enacted physical and/or sexual violence against an intimate partner, both over a lifetime and in the past year. The high prevalence of violence against women has been linked to gender beliefs, adverse experiences in childhood, psychological distress, and alcohol use among men. Cramped living conditions, and limited street lighting and public sanitation, meanwhile, are environmental factors that enable violence. The situation is exacerbated by ineffective and inefficient police action, which results in secondary victimisation for survivors and gives perpetrators a sense of impunity. The failings of the public sector to effectively address the drivers of violence and the needs of survivors have led to a number of NGOs (non-governmental organisations) developing prevention-and-response services to reduce violence against women. These include an organisation we refer to here as Bopelo ('life', a pseudonym), which has been working in Narrow Ridge to shift gender norms at the community level and encourage people to take action against violence against women. We illustrate this through the experiences of Lesedi and Siyabonga.

Lesedi is an African woman in her late twenties who grew up in a remote area of KwaZulu-Natal Province (KZN). Lesedi grew up on a remote farm, and spent much of her youth playing with brothers. By the time she went to university in the late 2000s, Lesedi had adopted a masculine style, developed a rough persona and for a while had relationships with women. However, in 2007 her father died and she met Thabo. She began to party a lot at university and did not get good grades. Eventually she dropped out. Soon after, in 2010, she became pregnant and had a baby boy, Karabo. Thabo began to consume drugs and started to physically abuse Lesedi. She fought back, but recognised the danger as Thabo's aggression increased as he consumed more drugs.

Lesedi decided to return home, and there she earned money by trading alcohol informally while her mother looked after Karabo. This allowed Lesedi to support her family financially and obtain some independence. Lesedi continued to see Thabo and, despite using condoms when they had sex, she became pregnant again in 2012. She went to live for a while with relatives far away from both Thabo and her mother and son, and unsuccessfully tried to have an abortion. She gave birth to a baby girl, Ntombi. Lesedi began to self-harm and destroyed everything Thabo had bought for her.

Lesedi returned to live with her mother and her two young children. She maintained the relationship with Thabo because he provided her with financial support. However, the money he gave her – around R600–R1 000 a month – was insufficient to cover groceries, clothes and nursery costs. Lesedi began to gamble in an attempt to increase the little money Thabo gave her. She also began to visit Thabo less, as his drug use and his aggression were increasing. Thabo was annoyed that Lesedi would not move in with him and would complain that she only visited him when he got paid. Fights would start when Thabo returned home late from work and demanded sex. Lesedi would complain that she was too tired from looking after the children, since she did not have the help of her mother, and this would enrage Thabo. One time he chased her, and the children, out of the house at 10 p.m. In an attempt to resolve their problems, they visited a social worker, but Thabo did not change and became increasingly controlling. He would phone Lesedi and make her leave her phone on so he could hear what she was doing; he would sit up all night on drugs and then go to work. In 2016, she ended the relationship, but she maintains contact with him out of fear that he will hurt their children. She moved to Narrow Ridge in search of work, leaving her two children in KZN with her mother, confident that a change of environment would be good for her.

She found it hard to adapt to life in Narrow Ridge, however, and was sick for two months after the move, which she thinks was due to air pollution. Lesedi felt 'street-smart' and able to recognise dangerous situations, but she was always scared in Narrow Ridge. Once she was violently attacked at a social gathering over a seemingly innocuous interaction, suggesting to her that people in Narrow Ridge were quick to resort to violence. Limited job opportunities meant that many women depended on men to provide for them, and were often in relationships where there is no love, like Lesedi's relationship with Thabo. This led some women to sell sex or have multiple boyfriends to cover all their financial needs (transport, rent, going out). The commodification of sexual relationships made it especially dangerous for Lesedi to go out at night. Men would approach her and offer to buy her drinks. If she accepted, the man would expect a sexual favour; if she refused they would try to force her. Lesedi felt that men had little else to do other than try to get the attention of women.

Lesedi initially stayed with a cousin, but wanted to live alone in order to assert her independence. So she rented her own space with money that her mother sent her each month. However, the money was only enough for rent, and she was unable to pay for clothes, food, electricity, phone credit, recreation or transport, or cover additional unexpected costs (medical, legal fees). Unable to find paid work, Lesedi moved again to live with her aunt, on whom she could rely for food.

One day Lesedi attended a workshop held by Bopelo. The facilitators talked about sexual harassment and the importance of condom use. When the facilitators asked if anyone was interested in joining the project as a volunteer, Lesedi was quick to sign up. She began participating in community-education activities. She was enthusiastic and excited by the work and felt that public speaking was something she was good at. Although she does not get paid, Lesedi appreciates that volunteering has given her something meaningful to do with her time, and it helps her to avoid drinking and smoking. In this role, she draws on her own experiences and advises people to leave abusive relationships. She explains how her desire to help Thabo overcome his problems, and her economic dependence on him, led her to be caught in a violent relationship for almost 10 years. If she were in the same situation now, she says, she would leave.

Siyabonga is a African man around 30 years old who was raised in a rural area of North West Province. After living in another of Johannesburg's townships, Siyabonga moved to Narrow Ridge in 2013 with his wife, while their children remained in the North West with his parents. Siyabonga was not comfortable moving to Narrow Ridge. He was frightened of the township's reputation for violence. People were always being mugged and having their cellphones stolen. He blames unemployment and drugs, such as *nyaope* – a cocktail drug, which includes antiretrovirals (ARVs) – as the causes of the high level of violence. Siyabonga also feels that the lack of electricity and street lighting enables crime and prevents people from having the freedom to walk at night. The maze of narrow streets in informal areas makes it easy for perpetrators to escape, and police rarely respond promptly to calls, if at all. He feels that men are responsible for most of the violence because they are the ones who take drugs. Theft is the only way to gain sufficient money to buy the expensive drugs they desire.

Siyabonga explains that men in Narrow Ridge are also violent to women. At night women are scared to go out in public, especially in areas that lack public lighting, for fear of being raped. They are also abused in their home by partners. Domestic violence, Siyabonga feels, is linked to socialisation. Drawing on his own experience, Siyabonga explains that boys in his home area are expected to run to the shop and buy groceries, and girls are expected to stay at home to cook, clean and wash. When he grew up, domestic chores were strictly for women, whereas men were supposed to go out into the world and provide. Siyabonga absorbed the idea that men were the household heads, with authority and decision-making power. When he married Joy, he believed that he should not have to answer to her, yet Joy should tell him everything. However, the legitimacy of Siyabonga's power over Joy was undermined by his inability to find work. Joy found employment and became the 'breadwinner'. Despite not contributing to the family finances, Siyabonga considered himself to be in sole charge of the money Joy earned. Unemployed, he would sit at home all day watching television and not do any housework. Joy would come home from a long day of work to his mess and dirty dishes. He would expect her to clean up, cook dinner, do the dishes, and then have sex with him. This created tension, led to arguments, and to Siyabonga physically assaulting his wife. She was like a punching bag, he explained, and he was hitting her 'like no-one's business'. He did not consider this abusive.

In the middle of 2016, Siyabonga attended a Bopelo workshop. He realised that his wife could lay a charge against him for abuse and he could be sent to prison. Siyabonga decided to volunteer and received training in facilitation. After participating in Bopelo's workshops, Siyabonga began to reconsider the gender norms he was socialised into. He now appreciates that Joy works hard and that there is no shame in a man washing, cleaning or cooking. He does not have to be forced to do domestic chores; he feels it is the right thing to do. The changes he has undergone have led Siyabonga to feel that participation in the Bopelo intervention is helping the community. It helps men like him recognise that they are abusive and to stop, while it helps women to understand their rights. As an example, Siyabonga explains how, during workshops, many people are unaware of the notion of sexual consent, and state that a husband cannot rape his wife; only strangers commit rape. Siyabonga feels that these assumptions highlight the lack of information about sexual violence, resulting in suffering and, on occasions, loss of life. Community education may not stop all violence, but Siyabonga believes it can reduce it by dispelling such myths and raising awareness of sexual consent.

Because of his personal experience of transformation, Siyabonga feels that community education can alter perceptions and reduce sexual violence. He has begun to talk to his friends about gender equality and share the knowledge that helped him to change his behavior. Volunteering with Bopelo, he says, has given him greater empathy for those around him and provided him with confidence to take action and intervene in situations where violence might occur; before he would not have done so. Siyabonga talks to his children about these issues. By washing, cooking and cleaning in front of his children, he challenges the social norms that he was brought up with. He believes that his children will learn from him.

Many people who migrate to urban areas in the search of waged labour find themselves living in informal housing, experiencing food insecurity, and under threat from violence. The threat of violence is felt most by women, who are vulnerable to both intimate-partner violence and to sexual assault in public spaces.

The high level of intimate-partner violence in Narrow Ridge is driven by individual men's adherence to patriarchal gender norms, which legitimise male-on-female violence within the household, and normalise it to the extent that physical and sexual assault is not considered abusive by the perpetrators. Violence is also fuelled by socioeconomic processes that generate endemic poverty and inequality. These factors deny working-class men the opportunity to obtain quality education, meaningful employment and the positive psychological benefits associated with these. Intimate-partner violence and other forms of violence against women in Narrow Ridge are further enabled by failings in the justice system and inadequate health services, which deny survivors of violence the support – such as shelter services, post-rape care, counselling and ongoing psychotherapeutic support – to leave abusive relationships. Together, these interpersonal, environmental and social determinants make violence an everyday reality for women living in communities like Narrow Ridge.

NGOs such as Bopelo are working to prevent and reduce violence against women by transforming how community members think about gender, and by encouraging them to take direct action against violence against women. However, the work of NGOs will only ever be part of the solution. Greater public investment in the physical and social infrastructure of Narrow Ridge is also needed, as are improvements to South Africa's education, health and justice systems, while a reduction in poverty and inequality is also necessary.

There is, we have noted, a growing number of female-headed households – either the household of a single woman and her dependents, or the multigenerational household with or without dependent young and elderly men as well as women. This should not imply that men are somehow adrift from households, or dissociated from the emotional, financial and social bonds that sustain them, or uninvolved in families and caregiving and its related labour (Morrell & Jewkes 2011). A growing number of men now maintain households as women migrate and find work, and are able to send cash remittances back home. Young men who cannot find employment on leaving school, and older men who have experienced long-term unemployment, also take on caregiving. The everyday responsibility for a household and care for individuals thus increasingly falls to any able-bodied person (see Block 2014, 2016; Block & McGrath 2019).

In this chapter, we have sought to extend our understanding of gender and masculinity beyond that which Robert Morrell, RW Connell and others refer to as hegemonic masculinity, and beyond its 'toxic' consequences in gender-based violence and sexual violence against women (Connell & Messerschmidt 2005; Davies & Eagle 2013; Jewkes et al. 2015; Luyt 2012; Morrell et al. 2012). By widening this lens, we have drawn attention to the complexity of households and families, as well as masculinities, men and women, in contemporary South Africa.

Note

1   The Mzantsi Wakho study combines qualitative and quantitative methods to investigate the health and social experiences of adolescents and young adults (N=1527 adolescents aged 11–19 in the baseline cohort). Established in 2013, the study is among the largest-known longitudinal, community-traced studies on medicines-taking and sexual health among HIV-positive adolescents.

5 Everyday care and illness

Lenore Manderson and Nolwazi Mkhwanazi

Families, as we have already noted, are dynamic, changing for multiple reasons: migration, health events, settlement, economic change, personal needs and interpersonal demands. Their membership expands around certain events, shrinks at other times. In this chapter, we turn from discussions of the roles of men and women in constituting, maintaining and nurturing families, to the role of families in providing care, both on an everyday basis and under exceptional circumstances.

Although we speak of families as genetically related, families are firstly networks of individuals through personal, not necessarily biological, relationships. Networks and relatedness do not depend on co-residence, and the care work conducted within families is largely work within households. This work is supplemented by others who move in or out of the household, or who contribute to the household in other ways, including financially or through regular communication, which today includes phone calls and WhatsApp messages as much as by visiting (Ahlin 2018).

How we conceptualise care, and describe its delivery in households, also varies by context. The care needs of infants or small children differ from the care needs and household tasks for older children and adults; the care needs of a child without health or developmental difficulties are quite different to those of children with problems in terms of mobility, learning or communication. Severity of impairment compounds the tasks of care. Likewise, the care delivered to and from adults within a house varies, both because the work of care is unevenly distributed through gender divisions and expectations, and because the health and wellbeing of individual members vary. Type of health problem further impacts what it means to care for and provide care practically; consider the different challenges associated with caring for people with mental-health problems, people with serious physical conditions that inhibit self-care, or people with a chronic degenerative disease. Ageing and frailty bring further complexity to care, as we shall explore in the following chapter.

A striking feature of discourses on care, and its provision by family members, is the implication that all members of a family care about each other, and so physical and other kinds of care – cooking, cleaning, assisting with self-care, and so on – are provided unproblematically and without stress. Discourses on the role of family members in providing care largely also assume that others in the household know how to care when care needs are complicated; for resource reasons especially, relatively little attention is paid to assisting people to learn to give care to those in need. Further, caregivers and care recipients are implicitly assumed to be separate categories, and overlaps between who is cared for and who is in need of care are ignored. But at any time, a person who is responsible for care – preparing meals, washing clothes, cleaning the house/yard, reassuring others – may also be in need of care, either for an acute or an ongoing health problem. Moreover, people rarely have one moment when they might need special support and care. Some care needs are lifelong; others are intermittent; some are temporary and bounded; many overlap.

The physical environment in which the majority of South Africa's population lives impacts health and wellbeing. The quality and materials of housing, determined by what families can afford to build or rent, directly affect health and wellbeing. The quality of housing includes the number of rooms in a house, the number of inhabitants, and the spaces and facilities to cook, bathe and sleep, and for children to do homework. Building materials may compromise mood, sleep patterns, and health; consider the high ambient temperatures in summer, and extreme cold in winter, in houses with both roofing and walls made of unlined tin. Townships, inner urban slums, informal settlements, gated communities, farms and villages provide families with different infrastructure and environments for living. Among these, we include the availability or absence of private or communal toilets, tap water and electricity (predictable or not), regular collection of rubbish, reliable and frequent transport systems, access to affordable food, employment opportunities, community safety and policing. The following all limit the capacity of householders to maintain their health: the poor quality of housing, crowding, limited external infrastructure and resources, and community disharmony. Keeping a house clean, for instance, is problematic if there is no access to water, or if the numbers of people living in the space make it almost impossible to stay on top of basic chores. Ensuring a healthy diet is problematic when fresh affordable food is not available locally, where home gardening is not possible, and where there is nowhere to store food in the house – as case study 4.3 by Rebecca Hodes illustrated. Focus on the household production of health needs to include the wider environment, for individual household capacity is seriously constrained when the environment is impoverished, and is immeasurably enhanced when the environment is health-giving, safe and clean.

In this context, the following case study (5.1) by Susan Levine, Alison Swartz and Hanna-Andrea Rother has particular relevance. Their departure point, on childhood poisonings, rests in part on Achille Mbembe's argument that under the effects of colonialism, capitalism and race, some humans are treated as 'waste'. This uncomfortable metaphor challenges environmental and public-health assumptions about the capacity to address the effects of toxic waste on human populations and within individual families, as if waste were separable from human experience. Waste is a problem at multiple levels: it includes human waste, and the measures needed to prevent contamination of humans by human waste; it includes waste generated through daily living, including left-over food and food packaging; it includes other rubbish that provides breeding grounds for rodents and cockroaches. Human health is compromised when waste cannot be managed. Mbembe draws attention to the ways that colonial public health dehumanised individuals, such that they assumed the status of waste, routinely regarded as surplus or disposable, and hence undeserving of protection from environmental harms. We would add to this insight the unrecognised role of waste pickers and night-soil and rubbish collectors, working individually or with local government, trying to manage environments that are increasingly unruly with growing population density and challenges of governance.

Case study 5.1 derives from a project in the School of Public Health and Family Medicine at the University of Cape Town, led by Hanna-Andrea Rother. The project involved research by anthropology and public-health students. Alison Swartz was part of the cohort of student researchers, and the case study draws on the data she collected in 2008 as part of her honours mini-dissertation (see Swartz et al. 2018 for a description of the research methods). The case study focuses on the use of agricultural pesticides, bought cheaply in unlabelled containers in unregulated markets, to protect children from rodent bites and exposure to other household pests. As the authors illustrate, children often consume the contents of such bottles, or eat foods accidentally contaminated by rat poison, or they are otherwise exposed to toxins, with life-threatening results.

Case study 5.1

The whistling of rats

Susan Levine, Alison Swartz and Hanna-Andrea Rother

> On that night she had been dreaming of a whistling sound. It was all around her. The whistling grew into a moaning. She opened her eyes but it was so dark that she couldn't see the ever-expanding belly of the ceiling, how it was creakily reaching towards her. But she heard, above the moaning, the frantic rats shrieking, hissing, swearing, chattering. (Miller 2016: 8)

Ma Taffy twitches at the thought of rats. Her ceiling houses an entire colony of rats. Before long 'rat shit started to drizzle around the house like a small, intermittent rain' (Miller 2016: 8). Ma Taffy lives in Jamaica, and she is a fictional character in Kei Miller's novel *Augustown*. Mama Kaya lives in South Africa, and she is not a fictional character. She also fears rats, and resents the conditions that draw rats into her home. The closer one gets to Mama Kaya's house from the main road in Lower Crossroads, the more chaotic the scene becomes, with narrowing streets full of potholes, untarred lanes, stagnant pools of water, and heaps of uncollected rubbish. A laundry line of children's faded clothes easily wrapped around Mama Kaya's house, which was flanked by a gradual, sandy slope decorated with rubbish and patchy yellow grass. Her house was made from bits of wood, metal and plastic, never quite upright, leaning against the next haphazard structure. The openings and leakages dissolved the boundaries between what was meant to reside inside and what was meant to reside outside, the threshold between home and the street too easily transgressed.

Our story opens in the children's poison unit at the Red Cross War Memorial Children's Hospital (RXH) in Cape Town, where Mama Kaya's daughter was being treated for organophosphate poisoning (OP). This ward was filled with doctors, nurses, cleaning staff and family caregivers, all expertly negotiating the limited space between the cots and the machines that beeped and telephones that rang above the hum of voices. In this setting, children's bodies were sites of pain and discomfort, weakness and poor motor control, but also sites where invasive medical equipment intervened.

Background

The Western Cape has a population of nearly six million, a growing number of whom live in low-income urban townships. Residents in both permanent and informal housing experience a range of environmental harms and health-related risks associated with poor sanitation, inadequate disposal of refuse, limited access to clean water, insecure housing, and pest infestation. To eliminate pests from domestic spaces, 'street pesticides' are used. The pests targeted include rodents and rodent fleas carrying diseases such as salmonella, leptospirosis and plague, and biting children and destroying food sources; cockroaches causing allergies and creating a stigma of uncleanliness; and other poverty-related pests, including flies, bedbugs and fleas (Rother 2008, 2010, 2016).[1] Street pesticides are unlabelled and illegal, and are sold by street vendors in plain containers or recycled bottles that once held juice, water or alcohol. Children mistake the contents of these containers as safe to consume (see Goldstein & Hall 2015).

Street pesticides are easily accessible and affordable in urban townships, and the demand for cheap and effective ways to eliminate pests keeps street-pesticide sellers buying, diluting and reselling agricultural pesticides. These pesticides usually have one active ingredient, or a mixture of active ingredients; these include methamidaphos, chlorpyrifos, cypermethrin or aldicarb. Aldicarb, for example, is used in agriculture to kill nematodes (that is, worms found in soil) and mites (for example, on potatoes, strawberries, and citrus), and is sold in strips of tiny black pellets. These ingredients were registered for agricultural use in food production when this research commenced in 2008 (Rother 2008), but, due to their extreme toxicity, they are not registered for domestic use by the South African Department of Agriculture under the Fertilizers, Farm Feeds, Agricultural Remedies and Stock Remedies Act (No. 36 of 1947). According to the WHO (World Health Organization) classification of acute hazards (WHO 2010), these substances range from being extremely hazardous to having limited acute hazards under normal-use conditions. Potential chronic health effects from exposure include neurotoxic, reproductive toxic and dermatoxic effects (that is, affecting the brain, reproduction and skin) and these may cause cancer (Roberts & Routt Reigart 2013; Rother 2008). Acute pesticide poisoning can result in drooling and runny noses, stomach pains, nausea, diarrhoea, vomiting, weakness, muscle twitching, headaches, confusion and, even, in severe cases, death. Long-term health effects include infertility and brain damage (Conant 2005).

Several cases on the ward

Mama Kaya's daughter Thandi, aged 12, reached for a bottle of drinking water, which was placed on a small, cluttered table next to her bed. The poison in the pale blue plastic bottle was invisible, and instead of quenching her thirst, Thandi had to be rushed to the RXH. Her mother had intended to use this mixture of pellets and water to keep her four children and grandchild safe from rats, and to keep her house cockroach free. The toxicity of the mixture could be clearly seen by damage to a blue wall in her small lounge area; the 'cockroach poison' had eaten the paint off the wall, much in the same way as it had eaten the inside of Thandi's gut and lungs.

In another hospital bed (a cot) lay a child named Mandy. Her small hands were bound in bandages to ensure that she would not hurt herself (if she had a seizure) or disturb the drip that snaked its way across her face and into her nose. The medical folder in the basket at the foot of her cot indicated that she had OP. Her mother Erica's face was drawn with exhaustion as she sat next to her four-year-old daughter.

Other women in the ward included the mothers of children from 8 months to 12 years, all being treated for poisoning. The women sat anxiously, speaking about their affliction as a single event folded into layers of misfortune, their children's suffering part of a broader fabric of exclusion and deprivation, sometimes to such an extent that the poisoning event itself was rendered less of a crisis than the conditions that produced it. Mandy's exposure to OP, for example, was due in part to living in a prefabricated wooden house in which a bare light bulb was pegged to blue plastic sheeting lining the makeshift ceiling. Upon the carpet-covered shelving, various crockery items and vases were neatly set out. The interior space suggested an intensity of care in cultivating an orderly domestic space, where Mama Erica pursued the preservation of life.

Mama Marcy, another participant in our study, explained how her three-year-old son had drunk 'the cockroach poison': 'There are bad cockroaches ... We are living next to dumps and it affects our places. We are fed up with cockroaches.' In Khayelitsha, the largest urban township in Cape Town, waste removal is unreliable, resulting in piles of rubbish being dumped near homes. The fierce winds of the Cape carry it through the township; it sometimes becomes caught in fences and windows, or banked up against home walls. Risk of poisoning is intensified by the insubstantial barriers of makeshift homes cobbled together with sheets of zinc, cardboard, old wooden planks, plastic sheets, random bricks and other found material. The daily injustices of poverty tie individual poisonings to the toxic layers of poverty and race oppression (Magubane 1979).

Other children in the poison unit had not been exposed to OP poisoning, but had come into contact with aldicarb. They included an eight-month-old baby boy. His mother, who attended to him closely for the five days he spent in the renal ward, explained that he had not even consumed the Aldicarb; rather, he had sucked on the packaging, a small crumpled piece of plastic that had contained the pesticide, before it was discarded. Another mother present had three-year-old twins, one of whom was in the hospital. He had eaten some adicarb-containing maize meal that had been placed on the floor. These women all explained how they mixed the small black granules of aldicarb with maize meal or bread, and then placed the mix in containers on the floor for rats and mice to eat. For curious and hungry children, the temptation to eat these mixtures was immense. The mother of the little twin described her fear that her son's body was going to bulge and distort itself in the same way that the bodies of rats poisoned with aldicarb do before they die.

According to Bernard Weiss (2000) from the Department of Environmental Medicine at the University of Rochester in New York, children are especially vulnerable to poisonings as they occupy a distinctive ecological niche in the world. Children spend much time on floors where toxic residues fall, and, as Weiss reminds us, 'Children literally lead a hand-to-mouth existence' (2000: 377). Entwined with these ordinary developmental stages, these children were also managing hunger. After consuming maize meal laced with aldicarb left under her bed, an eight-year-old girl explained, 'I was hungry.'

The effects of pesticide poisoning are not isolated. Instead, the poison circulates through children's body systems, resulting in multiple symptoms. Pesticide poisoning, and the contexts of poverty in which it occurs, blurs bodily boundaries, and children's health is overdetermined by intersections of hunger, pollution, poverty, immature biology, and shifting arrangements of care. Child pesticide poisoning exists in a crisis-filled landscape (London 2005).

Pesticides are all toxic; they are produced with the intention to harm. They are legislated for use within a government-defined framework of 'acceptable risks', but, as we have shown, street pesticides are a prime example of the layered toxicity of pesticides that result in unacceptable harms and unintended negative consequences. Rother has advanced numerous immediate interventions to combat these poisonings: through awareness campaigns, efforts to properly label illegal street pesticides, and the provision of alternative methods of control (rattraps for rodents, organic solutions to bed bugs, flies, and cockroaches). These public-health interventions are critical. However, historical inequalities set the stage for poisoning trauma, and these are folded in with the layers of waste that attract rodents to residential areas. Race and class oppression find their material moorings in the waste of old bed springs, mouldy mattresses, medicine packages, plastic bottles, torn shoes, cereal boxes, puddles of stagnant water, plastic bags and other domestic waste left to accumulate in heaps of hospitable mounds where rodents can prosper. As a result, residents in urban townships carry a dual burden of disease from exposures to pests and toxic pesticides (Rother 2010). To safeguard against infectious disease and to eliminate pests from domestic spaces, the women in this study did what they could to kill rats, mice and other pests. Here, paradoxically, cleanliness and childcare in the context of abject poverty are intimately linked to the purification of households with toxic poisons.

The state – the government of South Africa – takes on the responsibility to help to ameliorate some of the challenges that families face and that impact on household viability, family life, and the wellbeing of individuals. Poverty – through unemployment, insecure employment and low-paid jobs, food insecurity, the fragmentation of family systems, and increased care responsibilities – complicates the ability of women, especially, to provide family-based care of any kind. Caregiving is demanding, physically, financially and emotionally, and most caregivers provide care under stressful conditions, which in turn affects their mental wellbeing.

Cash-transfer programmes that the state has developed provide some support and enable resilience. The CSG, for example, aims to provide some income relief to poor families with children. But most families have very little support in caregiving, whether caregiving is defined in terms of providing householders with regular meals, or whether it is more complicated, for people unable to self-care. Case study 5.2 draws on data from intervention research conducted in Soweto and in rural Limpopo Province in 2016. Tessa Hochfeld, Jenita Chiba and Leila Patel focus on the experiences of female caregivers undertaking most of the domestic labour in their households. This case study describes a pilot preventive family-support programme with the goal of strengthening family functioning. The programme was concerned with women's ability to parent, with their everyday care and confidence in parenting, and with providing emotional support and guidance to their children.

Case study 5.2

Sihleng'imizi

Tessa Hochfeld, Jenita Chiba and Leila Patel

> Sometimes I wish they had a grandmother … maybe they will listen.
> Sometimes the kids are naughty and it's like I am alone because sometimes
> I am at work and sometimes I am doing night shift [so I am not there]. [I
> am trying to be a good mom] but I get frustrated when the children don't
> listen to me.

These words were shared by Thulani, aged 35 years, who is the daily caregiver for 4 children from 1 to 10 years old. She and her husband, the father of her children, live in a relatively well-serviced area in Soweto. He has a low-paid job, and she gets casual work in a factory when she can. She has a home with electricity, there are schools and clinics nearby, and she receives the CSG. However, caring for the children is not easy. Although she lives with her husband, she is solely responsible for the children's care. When she says 'I am alone,' she is referring to fulfilling her caregiver duties, which in South Africa are strongly gendered and considered women's work. While the state support is vital and having enough food to eat is critical, the long-term wellbeing of her children comes equally from the day-to-day love, warmth and consistency that she and others in her family offer them. Good caregiving is the key to how children build trust, mutuality, belonging and healthy relationships. The relationship between material, emotional and social care is complex, but all are critical in long-term positive outcomes for children (Patel et al. 2017a, 2017b).

With 55 per cent of South Africa's population living below the poverty line (Stats SA 2017), families in South Africa face many challenges, as has already been described. The CSG brings some income relief to poor families with children, despite its modest monetary value (R360/US$30 per month per child at the time of the study). The grant is largely spent on food and school-related costs. Other services, such as free primary healthcare, free education, the National School Nutrition Programme, and other provisions, complement the CSG by offering basic services to poor caregivers to support children's welfare. State and state-subsidised welfare and social-work services are limited in reach and delivery, and they are overloaded, offering interventions only at a point of crisis. Most families, therefore, have very little support beyond basic service delivery, which is patchy at best.

Poverty impacts significantly on caregiving, in ways that are sometimes surprising. For example, middle-class standards of monitoring young children are impossible when 'there is no dura hall [lock for the door] and no key at the gate [because I live in a backyard shack]. The kids just leave and you will look for them and it's not a playing issue [because of the dangers outside]' (Julia, aged 30 years, caring for 3 children – 11, 5 and 2 years old). Caregiving is also harder when there is overcrowding and a lack of safe spaces for leisure, when crime and violence are high, and when affordable quality childcare after school or for younger children is scarce. Nonetheless, despite poverty, children's long-term health and wellbeing is boosted significantly by growing up in a warm, loving home with committed, positive and consistent caregiving and positive role models. These aspects of caregiving are considered key 'protective factors' for risk behaviour and experiences, such as violence and child abuse, child mental illness, and social and behavioural problems (Berry & Malek 2017; Gorman-Smith et al. 2014; Meinck et al. 2015). While researchers have demonstrated positive outcomes of the CSG, including a moderate decrease in poverty (World Bank 2014) and improved school outcomes (attendance and number of years completed) (Heinrich et al. 2012), income support alone cannot lead to child wellbeing. Care – understood as the full range of physical care, 'caring about' and 'taking care of' children – plays a fundamental role alongside cash transfers in securing the current and future wellbeing of children in South Africa.

In 2016, a preventive family-intervention programme was piloted by the Centre for Social Development in Africa, University of Johannesburg, in two poor areas: Doornkop in Soweto and Moutse, a rural village in Limpopo Province. This programme was intended specifically to complement and scale up the positive impacts of the CSG, by offering a weekly meeting for 12 weeks for 4–6 families receiving 1 or more grants, facilitated by a trained social worker, to support the caregiving that the families currently provided to their children. Called Sihleng'imizi ('we care for families' in isiZulu), the programme aimed to strengthen family functioning in the following areas: child–caregiver relations; parental involvement in child's school; social and community connectedness; and financial literacy. A larger pilot and advanced testing using a quasi-experimental design was conducted in 2017; the results are currently being analysed.

Recruitment and sampling for the groups was via public primary schools in the research sites. Permission was sought from the school principal and the Provincial Department of Education. Children in Grade R (reception year, 5- and 6-year-olds) and Grade 1 (6- and 7-year-olds) who were receiving a CSG and displaying any behaviours of concern (such as being persistently late for school, or absenteeism) as identified by class teachers. The group facilitator explained the programme in detail in a home visit, and the whole family was invited to attend. The adult participants were primarily female caregivers; recruiting and retaining other adults, especially men, was a challenge. The ages of the children were from infants to teenagers, and parenting challenges of all ages were discussed in the group, although the programme focused primarily on middle childhood. Time limitations and work commitments prevented some families from participating, although they may have had other reasons too that they did not share. Four groups were run (two each in the urban and rural sites), with 100 per cent retention in three of the four groups.

The families gave permission for the pre- and post-intervention research, which evaluated the short- and medium-term effects of *Sihleng'imizi* qualitatively. There was also a six-month follow-up evaluation. The data illuminated the experiences of caregivers and their families, and the nature of care in poor families, and gave voice to how care contributes to the health and wellbeing of families and children. Two issues stood out. One was related to the social and community support critical for caregivers to have the personal and emotional means to provide care; the other was how being a loving caregiver can be undermined by a lack of appropriate caring skills. In all cases, caregivers were motivated to do the best for their family, and they attended *Sihleng'imizi* voluntarily. We describe these factors below, with quotations from primary caregivers who completed the *Sihleng'imizi* programme; their names have been changed.

Social and community support

Ubuntu is a widely celebrated notion of social care. Many South Africans consider ubuntu as a concept that is fundamental to society, and believe that the value underscores everyday life. This was our expectation, too, when we asked about social solidarity in poor communities. However, a social notion that is valued is not always practised, and the ideal and reality are often very different. Caregivers from the *Sihleng'imizi* intervention study spoke evocatively about the high levels of distrust and conflict in their communities, and how urbanisation means one cannot rely on neighbours or, even, family:

> In my community there is *nyaopes* [drug addicts]. They steal and do everything, you see. I cannot say I am 100 per cent safe ... [even] in my own yard with my kids, and 6 o'clock I am in the house [with the door locked because that is when it gets even more dangerous]. (Dineo, aged 39 years, cares for 3 children, aged 6 years, 4 years and 3 months)

> I do not trust [my neighbours]. When we got here we didn't know each other and now we don't really know each other actual names and we just call each other neighbour and they only know my nickname. (Lucy, aged 53 years, cares for her 2 grandchildren, aged 12 years and 7 years)

> I don't like my neighbours ... they have got stories [and gossip about me], I don't like them. I stay in my house with my kids ... I don't trust them. (Palesa, aged 32 years, cares for 5 children, aged 13 years, 9 years, 6 years, 20 months and 2 months)

One aim of *Sihleng'imizi* was to promote social and community connectedness via different processes. One process was to intentionally pair families living locally during the programme as '*Sihleng'imizi* Buddies'; another was to develop a norm in the group to share the successes and challenges of caregiving openly and in a supportive climate. This aim seemed to have a powerful impact on the kind of social and community support families were able to access after the group ended. Social isolation was far more prevalent than we expected in a community that espoused the notion of ubuntu, but was relatively easily broken via a purposeful and positive shared experience of *Sihleng'imizi*. The point was not just to form friendships, although this was potentially beneficial, but to form relationships that could support positive caregiving. Some comments (below) that illustrate the benefits specifically mention how these connections could be used to discuss their children and caregiving, whether positive or negative:

> It has helped me and by attending *Sihleng'imizi* things changed because I find that everyone was friendly and because since I had lost my parents I was just living my own life, washing dishes and staying at home, I no longer had friends. But this changed when I started at *Sihleng'imizi*, when I'm with those people my life changes a lot because they were friendly and you are able to talk with them as they don't have any problems ... I will be visiting them and some of them I know they stay around Snake Park, I just wanted them to give me directions [on looking after my children]. (Phutuma, aged 36 years, cares for 2 children, aged 7 years and 21 months)

> It has changed a lot because when I have problems that I can't talk about with my parents or [other people] about, I can chat to her and she will give me some advice, and if she has a problem as well she comes to me. (Nomsa, aged 23 years, cares for 2 children, aged 6 and 3 years)

> I will keep my relationships with my group members as we used to spend time and talk at *Sihleng'imizi*. It helped us a lot, so I was the kind of person who would say I'm not after friends but *Sihleng'imizi* taught me I can make friendships and have buddies, so I love my buddies, even now anytime I can go see and chat about our children and how life is going. (Ma Ntutu, aged 58 years, cares for 5 foster children, 1 aged 14 years, 1 aged 11 years, 2 8-year-olds, and a 6-year-old)

Even without formal follow-up with these families, their relationships have continued over time, as we learned in a subsequent set of interviews, when women spoke, six months post-intervention, of continued relationships and support. Even without longer-term data, this aspect of the programme had an important immediate outcome, with positive social networks and relationships able to support families living in tough circumstances. Being socially connected enables young people to participate in activities that strengthen their relations with their peers and communities, builds resilience and gives a sense of belonging. Social connectedness – of the right kind – also protects children (Synergos 2014: 2).

Caring skills

Another issue *Sihleng'imizi* aimed to address related to the process and practice of discipline of children. As we have mentioned, caregivers took part voluntarily in *Sihleng'imizi*, and they were motivated to invest positively in their families. In all cases they wanted the best future possible for their children.

The majority shared the most common form of discipline in their homes: physical punishment (smacking or hitting). African families are traditionally authoritarian, and children are expected to comply with adults' expectations unquestioningly. Adults in the programme had commonly experienced corporal punishment in their own homes as children, and, despite its proscription by law, it is largely what parents know. Yet a few simple skills in alternative forms of discipline seemed to have major impact on how caregivers managed children's behaviour.

Participants' comments reflect these changes:

> I would like to say that ever since I started with this programme, discipline meant something in my understanding and not what I have learned it to be. First of all, from how we were brought up, there was a strong belief that a child will only understand or hear better if they are disciplined and that discipline meant beating, harsh, harsh discipline. Before coming here, I also believed that for a child to hear what you want to say and if not adhering to what you say, the only solution was to mete out harsh punishment, discipline and that meant giving a child a hiding. I have learned that discipline in a form of beating a child is not 'the' way but there are many other ways that you can give as means of disciplining a child. (Lindi, aged 68 years, caring for her 4 grandchildren, aged 12, 9, 8 and 6 years)

> I don't punish them [with a smack anymore]. They taught us at *Sihleng'imizi* that if a child does something naughty, they taught us a method called 'cool down', that is when they stand against the wall and hold it and not watch the TV as I know that is what he likes, as others watch he knows he's not allowed to watch because he has been naughty [so this has made him change more than the smack]. (Ma Ntutu, aged 58 years, cares for 5 foster children, aged 14 years, 11 years, 2 8-year-olds, and a 6-year-old)

> I bought some stickers that says good luck and they tell me everything so when he does something I give him a star sometimes, sometimes I give him one rand then he will go and change it and put it in his savings, so at least he gets some rewards. (Nomsa, aged 23 years, cares for 2 children, aged 6 and 3 years)

> At first I used to beat her but after attending at the *Sihleng'imizi* programme they told me that beating a child is not the right thing to do and it's better to give her a five-minute count down so that she can keep quiet in that five minutes, and from then I could see that she is starting to change and she is listening more. (Phutuma, aged 36 years old, cares for 2 children, aged 7 years and 21 months)

> The family is a primary and most important space of care, and state services cannot substitute for the social and emotional care delivered by families and communities. But child wellbeing is complex, and income support cannot claim to deliver it in its entirety. This is all the more reason to recognise how one promotive and preventive family programme can have significant positive effects on children in the longer term, and complement the CSG. Providing the opportunity to create positive and supportive social networks, and offering caregivers some simple skills to better manage their children's behaviour, can go a long way to better outcomes for child wellbeing.

Tessa Hochfeld, Jenita Chiba and Leila Patel have described in case study 5.2 an intervention to support women, relatively isolated by poverty and the demands of caring for middle-age children, an age group that has attracted limited attention in the scholarly literature and policy (however, see Mkhwanazi et al. 2018). In contrast, much has been written on adolescence. It is characterised everywhere as a time of physiological, neurocognitive, and socio-emotional changes, when young people may desire and seek to establish greater autonomy over their daily lives, pushing against – and yet still in need of – caregiving structures and the imperatives of love and support. Young people seek to make their own decisions about choices of friends and activities, and their sexual and reproductive behaviours, within the bounds of what is morally sanctioned, permitted or demanded by adults around them, including parents, other caregivers, relatives and friends. At the same time, the caregiving structures and caregiving practices in place – including the residential household and family network – mediate young people's access to resources, including food, clothing and other daily needs, material goods, support to attend school, and healthcare services. In order to exercise greater autonomy, including in sexual relationships, adolescents may risk losing access to the moral and physical support provided within their households, but they may also tap into other resources.

In the following case study (5.3), drawing on research conducted in the Eastern Cape, Rebecca Hodes, Beth Vale and Elona Toska explore the complex interplay of caregiving structures and practices, on the one hand, and sexual health outcomes among adolescents, on the other. The authors draw on data from research conducted for the Mzantsi Wakho project (see Chapter 4) through observations, interviews and focus-group discussions. In this case study, they focus on how HIV positive adolescents may experience greater stigma and discrimination within and by association to households, and be subject to greater surveillance regarding sexual practices, particularly because their HIV status marks these practices as dangerous. By contrasting young people's accounts of their experiences, we see how adult caregivers and adolescents understand and enact care and control within a nexus of intimate relationships.

Case study 5.3

The *mis*closure of an adolescent's HIV status

Rebecca Hodes, Beth Vale and Elona Toska

With the global move towards 'test and treat', the goal of HIV-testing programmes is to initiate all who test HIV positive onto antiretroviral treatment (ART) as rapidly as possible, ideally at the same session at which they test HIV positive. Because effective treatment results in viral suppression, HIV transmission is rare among those who are stable on medicines, hence the phrase 'treatment as prevention'. However, parallel with evidence about the health benefits of HIV testing, HIV-status knowledge and ART initiation, questions have arisen about the potentially negative consequences of HIV status disclosure (Granich et al. 2009). With such large-scale testing and treatment campaigns underway, in varied contexts and among diverse populations, is it a certainty that telling someone that they are HIV positive will benefit their health and enable them to adhere to medicines and use condoms during sex?

Beginning in 2013, the study on which we draw began to focus on the significance, for adolescents, of being told that they were HIV positive. We explored the outcomes of HIV disclosure on adolescents' healthcare behaviours, specifically adherence to antiretroviral (ARV) medicines (Cluver et al. 2015) and their use of condoms to protect against HIV transmission (Toska et al. 2015). We found that knowledge of an adolescents' own HIV status was strongly associated with safe sexual practices. Thus, if they knew that they were HIV positive, they were more likely to report that they had used condoms during sex. However, disclosing their HIV-positive status to a sexual partner was not associated with a reduction of unsafe sex. Interviews helped to qualify and explicate these findings and unravel the consequences of HIV disclosure for individual adolescents. The interviews were located in adolescents' homes and leisure spaces, rather than in healthcare facilities in which young people are on their best behaviour (Vale et al. 2017). Below, we explore an instance of *mis*closure, in which disclosure of HIV status to a teenager resulted in negative consequences for her health.

Dineo's defaulting

Dineo was interviewed four times between August and December 2014, three times in her home and once in the paediatric ART ward of a hospital. In 2014, Dineo was 15 years old. She had been HIV positive since birth, and had been initiated onto ART in 2008. The third of the four interviews with Dineo was conducted with her best friend and neighbour, Alicia, whom an interviewer described as her 'partner in crime'. In the weeks prior to the first interview, Dineo and Alicia were alleged to have taken their caregivers' social grant cards, drawn money intended for the family's subsistence for the coming month, and gone 'out partying'. According to their caregivers, they had spent the stolen money on alcohol and had not returned home for a number of days, their whereabouts unknown. Neither Dineo nor Alicia spoke about this in their conversations, but during one visit to their home, passing neighbours shouted at Dineo and Alicia and told the interviewer that the girls were 'out of control'.

Dineo's grandmother, Ezzy, in her mid-sixties, was interviewed twice during the same period. Dineo and Ezzy had differing accounts of Dineo's HIV disclosure and defaulting, but with a shared contention: Dineo's HIV disclosure was a pivotal event in her adherence to HIV medicines. She had been told by an uncle that she was HIV positive at age 11 as a warning against bad behaviour, but the *mis*closure had the opposite effect. Dineo's risk behaviours amplified; her ART adherence worsened.

Ezzy's view

Ezzy is Dineo's maternal grandmother. She has taken care of Dineo since she was just a baby. Before Ezzy became her formal guardian, Dineo was staying nearby with her mother, Patti, and father. Ezzy did not like Dineo's father as he used to hit her mother, and she urged Patti to come home to stay with her and leave Dineo's father. Patti refused. After Dineo was born, Ezzy heard stories from community members that Patti was not taking good care of her. This included leaving Dineo alone while she (Patti) went out partying.

Dineo's father became ill with TB, and he died a few weeks later. Then Patti came back home, also in poor health. Ezzy did not know anything about their HIV status, but she had heard rumours that both of Dineo's parents had 'AIDS'. A few days after Patti moved in, she became very sick. She was admitted to a local hospital and was put on a drip. The following day Ezzy went to visit Patti and asked the nurse if they had found out what was wrong with her. The nurse told her to ask Patti; they had told her. Patti revealed to Ezzy that she had been told by the nurses that her HIV test had returned positive, but she rejected this, insisting that she had only been with one man, Dineo's father, and that he had died from TB, not HIV. Patti was discharged and was doing well, but she began to use alcohol and ignored Ezzy's pleas to take care of her health. Patti started to get sick again and was readmitted to hospital. During this stay at the hospital, Ezzy helped with the care of Patti, taking night shifts so that she could be near her, and helping nurses to change, feed and care for her. Before Patti died, she asked forgiveness from Ezzy.

Ezzy was heartbroken. She told herself that she would make sure Dineo survived 'this disease', and asked God to give her strength.

After Dineo's mother's death, Ezzy started taking care of Dineo, who was about two years old at the time. Dineo was healthy until, in early 2008, she started to get sick. She began to take 'her pills' (ARVs) in late 2008, although she did not know what they were for. Ezzy said that, while growing up, Dineo did not give her problems with taking her pills: 'She [Dineo] was used to it. It was a fun thing to do, and she liked the attention she got when reminded to take her pills.'

In 2010, hospital staff asked Ezzy when she planned to tell Dineo that she was HIV positive. Ezzy said she would, but needed time to prepare herself. She then told Dineo's uncle that his niece had HIV.

Dineo had started playing on the streets until late in the evening, and because it was the time of the (soccer) World Cup, Ezzy and Dineo's uncle did not mind. But slowly, Dineo's behaviour started to change, and coming home late became more frequent, even after the World Cup. Ezzy complained to Dineo's uncle that Dineo no longer listened to her. Angered by his niece's behaviour, Dineo's uncle came to speak with her. In the course of their conversation, he told her that she should not be going out at night because she was sick with HIV.

Dineo later asked Ezzy what her uncle had meant. Ezzy told her then that that she had contracted HIV from her mother. Dineo asked whether that was what had caused her mother's death. Ezzy confirmed this, but added, 'Because you are taking your pills now, you will not be sick and you will live a long life until God decides to take you.' Ezzy explained that the pills were needed for the rest of her life and she must never miss them, or she would become sick and die. The next time she took Dineo to the hospital, for a repeat dose of HIV medicines, she asked the doctor to speak to Dineo about her HIV status and the importance of taking her pills. Dineo began to ask questions about what she had heard about HIV at school, including that many young people had died from the virus. Ezzy reported that since the disclosure of her HIV status, Dineo had stopped taking her pills.

Dineo's view

Dineo was shy and reticent in interviews. The young female interviewer, part of the team, proceeded cautiously, fearing crossing the line between an interview and an interrogation. Dineo lived in a shack, with little room for private conversations. In interviews, the researcher would suggest that they go for a walk or sit outside, out of earshot of family members, while other researchers – an older woman and a young man – talked with her aunt in their living room. Dineo's own reports of adherence were inconsistent. In single interviews, she would claim that she never missed doses, but also that she had missed pills the previous week. Her reports of using condoms during sex were similarly inconsistent. In the course of the study, Dineo's health worsened and she was hospitalised. Dineo requested that researchers visit her in hospital, where she stayed for some weeks, to help relieve boredom. At this point, she had not taken HIV treatment for about three months.

When recalling the various, haphazard conversations entailed in learning her own HIV status, Dineo said of her grandmother: 'She told me I was infected by my mom when she was breastfeeding me.' Interviewers asked whether Dineo had understood what her grandmother was telling her. She responded that she had, because of a conversation she had previously with her uncle. She explained that because her uncle believed she was dating, he had disclosed her HIV status to her, as a means of curtailing her behaviour: 'He told me I was HIV and to take care of myself. He was telling me to behave myself. Then I told him that I will never date.' Dineo said her uncle had explained the dangers of dating and of being on the streets at night, including the risks of rape. Researchers asked Dineo if she had known what HIV was when her status had first been disclosed to her. She responded that she had known, since she had been told that her uncle was himself HIV positive: 'She [my grandmother] told me my uncle have "this thing".' Dineo believed her uncle had been cured of HIV, but that he did not wish to share the cure with her.

Misclosure

Dineo's uncovering of her HIV status was not a textbook disclosure, carefully facilitated by family and health providers. Increasingly, the literature on adolescent HIV reports that disclosure, rather than being a one-off event, unfolds as a process, shaped by caregivers' fears regarding its consequences for the health and wellbeing of adolescents and other family members (Bikaako-Kajura et al. 2006; Kidia et al. 2014; Mattes 2014). Ezzy, for example, believed she needed more time to 'prepare herself' before disclosing Dineo's HIV status to her; disabusing her granddaughter of various 'protective deceptions' – including the causes of her parents' death, and the purpose of her chronic medicines – would bring Ezzy pain. And she feared the consequences for Dineo's health, which she had undertaken to protect. In the interim, the responsibility for guarding Dineo's knowledge about her own HIV status, while ensuring that she remained adherent to HIV medicines, was primarily Ezzy's.

Dineo's discovery of her HIV status involved multiple people and institutions: her uncle, her grandmother, her school, her doctor and her nurses. Some of what she heard positioned HIV as a deadly virus, from which her mother had died. Additional information suggested she could live a long, healthy life with HIV, through diligent pill-taking. Complicating this were the pieces of information she had received and inferred about her uncle's HIV status, which suggested a possible cure. At the very least, it seemed to Dineo that her uncle's HIV status had not entailed the same moral and behavioural burdens as her own.

In learning of her own HIV status, Dineo was also required to recast her previous years' pill-taking, her mother's death, and her relationship with her grandmother, who had withheld pieces of these narratives. Our research suggests that for many orphaned, perinatally infected adolescents, ART adherence is inextricably bound up with remaking their deceased mothers' memories and suturing intergenerational ties (Vale & Thabeng 2016).

The multiple, at times contradictory, narratives that adolescents like Dineo receive about their HIV status can foster doubts and suspicions, including how HIV is transmitted and is treated. In Dineo's case, this revealed itself most strongly in her belief that her uncle had a 'cure' for HIV that he was not willing to share, and that he was wielding his knowledge of her HIV status to control her behaviour.

By Dineo's account, her uncle's disclosure of her HIV status had taken a punitive edge, in which he attempted to frighten her into behaving better. While her past pill-taking had reportedly been associated with positive recognition and attention from her grandmother, through this *mis*closure, HIV and its treatment had taken the form of reprimand and reprisal.

Dineo was not the only adolescent participant in our study who associated the discovery of her HIV status with attempts by her family to exert greater controls over sexual behaviours. The HIV status of a number of participants, principally young women, had been revealed in struggles with their guardians to 'bring them under control' – back into alignment with proscriptions of health and decency. In some instances, these adolescents had sought compensatory validation and acceptance outside their homes, including from sexual partners. The rejection of treatment by Dineo and others served also as a rejection of their family's admonishments, and as an assertion of greater bodily and sexual autonomy.

Current practices and recommendations of HIV status disclosure for children and adolescents living with HIV assume that age-appropriate, incremental knowledge-sharing from healthcare providers and caregivers will result in positive health outcomes. Case study 5.3 illustrates the tensions and doubts that shared knowledge of HIV status may bring. The disclosure of an adolescent's HIV-positive status may not always be conducted in a coordinated fashion, especially when multiple caregivers – including relatives and healthcare workers – are involved. For adolescents who have been HIV positive since infancy, revelations of their own status are related to new understandings about the legacies of their parents, and to its implications for their own lives and futures.

HIV testing, status disclosure, and treatment initiation are the bases of the global AIDS response. Public testing and treatment programmes account for many of the gains in HIV-related morbidity and mortality. Knowing that one is HIV positive, and understanding that one needs chronic medicines for health and survival, is an assumed prerequisite for effective HIV treatment among adults. But how does this apply to HIV-positive children and adolescents? How can they be tested, 'disclosed to' and treated, when often they have been diagnosed in infancy or early childhood, when their awareness of their status is preceded by the knowledge of many others, and when they have already been taking HIV treatment for many years?

Anna Versfeld, in the following case study (5.4), is concerned with the impact of adult ill health on families, and with how the state can provide care and support resilience. When health problems require the hospitalisation of a caregiver, then the welfare and wellbeing of others are inevitably unsettled. But in the cases she describes, the underlying causes of ill health are also care related: the women's use of methamphetamine was linked to their own efforts to self-care and to care for others, and to maintain their families. One of the two women in this case study, Shireen, explained her methamphetamine use as a measure to maintain her relationship with her husband. The other woman, Babalwa, used the drug to cope with depression. The women were not hospitalised with methamphetamine use, however, but rather with health problems that flowed from it and that they related to it: tuberculosis and HIV.

Shireen and Babalwa were both admitted to DP Marais Tuberculosis Hospital in Cape Town, desperately ill with tuberculosis and uncontrolled HIV. Because of their hospitalisation – four months for Shireen, six months for Babalwa – their young children were placed in state foster care. Although this has the potential for disastrous outcomes, in these cases, through a combination of state support processes – hospitalisation, temporary foster care for their children, and social-grant and housing provision – both women were able to stabilise and recraft their lives and families on hospital discharge. Informed by a hospital ethnography and interviews with men and women with TB, Versfeld illustrates how substance use may be the stuff of both social connection and disconnection, and how vital state support is to stitching together fractured families, even if that support requires the temporary splitting of the family unit.

Case study 5.4

Catching women before they fall out of the world

Anna Versfeld

Prior to the discovery of effective treatment for tuberculosis in the mid twentieth century, bed rest and fresh air were frequently prescribed as the best chances of cure, with tuberculosis sanatoriums providing these perceived healing elements. With the discovery of a relatively effective antibiotic cure for tuberculosis, sanatoriums – architectural reminders of a plague past – declined internationally (Bates 1992; Rothman 1995). However, countries with a high burden of HIV, such as South Africa, have seen a spike in tuberculosis infection, and public tuberculosis hospitals continue to play a fundamental role in efforts to contain the disease, providing housing and care for people who are too sick, or do not possess the resources, for curative healing at home. Cape Town has two such facilities, Brooklyn Chest Hospital and DP Marais TB Hospital. The two facilities house some 500 people at any one time. Approximately two-thirds are infected with HIV. At DP Marais, over half were identified as using substances (drugs and alcohol) when they became sick with tuberculosis (Versfeld 2017).

Shireen and Babalwa, aged 35 and 40 respectively, were both admitted to DP Marais, desperately ill, in early 2015. I met them both in a support group for people who used substances. The meeting was held in the 'sewing room', although the room was no longer used for sewing – the machines were all broken. Rather, it was a place where women who were in hospital for extended periods could earn extra income through activities such as ironing staff members' laundry or organising the folders of medical records for incoming patients. Shireen's third internment had lasted for four months. Babalwa's first lasted eight months, the duration of her treatment for disseminated tuberculosis. The women came from opposite parts of the country, spoke different languages, and had been, under apartheid, differently classified – Shireen 'coloured', Babalwa 'African' – and so they were differently treated by the state until 1995. They had limited interaction while moving through the same spaces in the hospital, but their journeys into, through and out of the tuberculosis hospital connect in multiple ways. This is the story of their lives, those connections, and the role of skeleton state support in catching marginalised women and families.

Shireen

Shireen was born and raised in a suburb developed during apartheid for people classified as coloured. She was raised by her mother and stepfather, who both worked in the hotel trade – her mother as a waitress, her stepfather as a barman. Her childhood was, as she described it, relatively stable, despite the constraints and difficulties of a working-class family at the time. At 16, she left school, she explained, to try to assist her parents by generating an income. At 18, she became pregnant from the young man with whom she was living in a rented room. When she was heavily pregnant, she looked on as her boyfriend was shot dead on their doorstep in a gang-related incident. Unable to manage on her own, after giving birth she sent her daughter to live with her paternal grandparents. Shireen met another man, continued working, and bore two more children. This relationship ended when her biological father extracted her and the children from the domestic violence they were suffering, and they went to live with him in a small, desolate, industrial town – Atlantis – some 130 kilometres out of Cape Town. There, Shireen found work and relative contentment. Her entertainment, like that of many around her, often consisted of drinking to the point of drunken slumber.

About a year after she had moved, Shireen was woken by her father's sexual advances. She packed up her children and returned to Cape Town to live with her mother and stepfather. While she described her stepfather as a decent man (on the basis, she explained, that he never abused her), she felt as though she was carrying an unfair burden of the household work – there were a number of younger sisters. She left to stay in a rented room. A year later, she moved into a shelter, but accommodation was contingent on abstinence from alcohol. Shireen was caught drinking one night and summarily dismissed from her home. From there, she relied on various friends for accommodation until she met Amin, the man she would later marry. Amin was already a father of two, and when Shireen became pregnant by him, he left her and returned to the mother of his children. A week before she gave birth he returned to her. They were married two weeks later, and had two more children.

Amin did not drink; he smoked methamphetamine. On the weekends, when he had been smoking (with other women) and Shireen was drunk, they fought. Amin had quick fists. Seeking a smoother relationship, Shireen switched from drinking alcohol to methamphetamine. She and Amin started to smoke together. They didn't need much, she said, just two packets to last them both for the weekend; Amin kept their use consistent and weekend bound. Shireen's substance switch was a strategic decision, and the fighting abated.

About two years later, Shireen started coughing and struggling to breathe. Amin frequently called an ambulance for emergency oxygen. In the months that followed, weight melted off her; eventually, she stopped smoking methamphetamine. However, after two weeks, things were no better. 'I still looked like a person who was smoking, even though I wasn't,' Shireen explained. She sought healthcare beyond the short-term oxygen provided by emergency ambulance services. She was diagnosed with tuberculosis and admitted to DP Marais Hospital, where she received treatment, food and shelter, and was able to rest. After two months, she took leave from the hospital to collect the grant (Child Support Grant) provided for her children. She did not return and her treatment lapsed.

Months later, she was returned into care involuntarily by ambulance services. She stayed for four months, but after going to her mother's funeral she did not return. Shireen explained these hospital departures in a number of ways, varying from 'It wasn't my time [to be healed],' to 'That was caused by the methamphetamine,' and her husband's resistance to her being away and leaving the children with him. The third resurgence of tuberculosis led to the hospitalisation during which we met. This time Shireen stayed in the hospital until the end of her treatment period. Her youngest three children were placed in foster care.

Shireen's treatment was fairly straightforward in biomedical terms. She restarted antretrovirals (ARVs) for HIV and became healthier; her viral load decreased. She responded well to tuberculosis treatment. By the end of her treatment, she was spending most days in the laundry room, ironing to generate some income. There she excitedly, proudly, told me (and anyone else who would listen) that she had a new house – a government-provided house in a new area. She was, she said, selected by the housing committee in the area where she had lived to be the recipient due to her illness. The government had provided a location and basic materials, and her husband had built it. Shireen left the hospital to move into her new home.

Babalwa

Babalwa's referral letter described a litany of health issues, including HIV, a productive cough and constitutional symptoms for TB: dysentery, wasting, fevers and chronic headaches. It also included a 'social' reason for admission to DP Marais: 'Hx [history] non-adherence.' Over the page, a second note read: 'Patient at high risk of defaulting, needs placement at DP Marais ...'

Babalwa was kept in the hospital until the end of her tuberculosis treatment. During this period, she religiously attended the substance-(ab)use awareness sessions in the hospital, although as an isiXhosa first-language speaker with limited English, she clearly could not always follow the conversations. No matter what the question, she would sit forward nervously, rub her hands up and down her thighs, and express much the same sentiment: 'I want to leave the bad things I was doing. I want to be a mother and father to my children because I don't have any family ...' Wendy, the group coordinator, would ask the same question of her, again, louder. Babalwa's response, a self-pleading, was unchanged: 'I want to leave the bad things I was doing, I want to be a mother and father to my children because I don't have any family ...'

Babalwa was born in the late 1970s in the Transkei, an area designated a Xhosa 'homeland' by the apartheid government. Most families relied on wage remittances from migrants working in the South African labour system. Babalwa lived with her parents until she was three years old, when both were killed in murders related to accusations of witchcraft. Her grandmother raised Babalwa, until she passed away when Babalwa was in her late teens.

Bereft and without family ties on which she felt she could draw, Babalwa went to seek a living and a life in Cape Town. She stayed with a friend in a township distant from the city centre. Unable to find work, her friend advised her to find a boyfriend, who could, at least, buy her toiletries. This she did; not long afterwards, she became pregnant and gave birth to a son. Her boyfriend was involved in crime. After some violence, fearing for her life, Babalwa fled with her baby back to the Eastern Cape. But life was no more sustainable there. Desperate, she returned to Cape Town to seek work; this time she was successful, finding employment in a factory. She struck up a new relationship, which was steady until she became pregnant again, approximately five years after her first child had been born. The pregnancy rocked the relationship – her partner did not want her to keep the child. He gave her R500 to have an abortion. She abandoned the plan ('It is my blood!' she explained to me), kept the child, bought food with the money, and remained steadfast in her choice. In order to hide her swelling belly, she stopped work and returned to the Eastern Cape, only returning to Cape Town late in her pregnancy when it was clear for all to see and too late for a termination. Her partner refused to support her, and the relationship ended. Deeply unhappy, she started to drink and continued to drink heavily through the rest of pregnancy. By this time, she had acquired HIV. However, she was on state-provided ARVs at the time of the birth, and although her daughter was breach – which Babalwa blamed on her drinking – she was born HIV negative.

After the birth, Babalwa and her children lived in a shack on the sandy margins of the city. She tried to survive by paying for rent and food with the little money she received from CSGs. This did not stretch to food for herself. She stopped taking her ARVs, which require food in the stomach, and staved off the worst hunger pangs by drinking water. In July 2013, the depths of winter, Babalwa, with a baby of two months old, found out that she had tuberculosis. In August, her own food ran out completely and with it her ability to produce breastmilk. Her baby started to starve, too. In September, aware she was dying, she called her uncle in the Eastern Cape. In describing her own potential death to me, she used the word *ukufa*. This is the Xhosa word used to describe the death of an animal, not a person. The word encapsulates the process of dying without dignity. In late September, when Babalwa was sick almost to death, a neighbour called an ambulance. Babalwa was driven to Groote Schuur Hospital, one of the largest specialist public hospitals in the city. Her baby, who had diarrhoea and vomiting, was taken to Red Cross Children's Hospital. From Groote Schuur, Babalwa was taken to DP Marais, with a diagnosis of disseminated tuberculosis. Her children were taken into state custody and put into foster care.

Better endings

As far as I was able to follow them, both women's stories had relatively positive endings. By the time of their departure, illness was not visible in either woman. Both had spent as much time as possible generating income through working in the sewing room once they were healthy enough. Babalwa saved the income from her grants and the ironing work to rent a small shack and re-forge her family. She kept in touch with a member of the occupational-therapy team, who paid her occasionally to come in and clean her house. She had her children back, she was not drinking, and she was doing well.

A few weeks after Shireen's discharge, I wended my way along a rough track to a crop of shiny-new tin shacks perched on a bluff, overlooking the ocean. Shireen's home was crowded by a single bed pressed into the corner, a plastic white chair that also served as a bedside table, a small kitchen table and a cupboard. The one small window sat so high it framed only blue sky; the open door let in light. But it was a home, and Shireen was proud of it. The final, extended, stay in hospital, when she had not used methamphetamine, combined with having a new home, allowed her to reconstitute her identity as a 'respectable mother' (Salo 2003), and away from drug dealers, Shireen explained, she reshaped life.

Both women's lives demonstrate the extreme vulnerability of women to sexual and physical violence within the home, the discombobulation of poor families in South Africa, and the ways in which poor health is situated in poor social conditions. These life narratives further illustrate how substance use may be the stuff of both social connection and disconnection. Methamphetamine use improved the relationship between Shireen and her husband, but ultimately compounded her poor health, her multiple hospitalisations, and the removal of her children into foster care. For Babalwa, alcohol provided a small escape from very difficult circumstances, but it also contributed to her illness, her hospitalisation, and six months of separation from her children.

In situations of marginalisation, the limited state support – mostly only supplied in post-apartheid South Africa – provided a critical net, catching these women before they fell out of the world. Both women relied on and used CSGs for survival, ambulances, and a public healthcare system through which they could be hospitalised (at no cost to them) to pull them back from the illness precipices over which they could easily have tipped. The provision of ARVs, hospitalisation, foster care for their children, CSGs, and access to housing – shacks – on discharge, allowed both women to find stability and to recraft their lives and families. In the short term, marginalisation fractured their lives, and state support required the separation of these mothers and their children. In the long run, however, limited state support provided essential family sustenance and suturing.

HIV features in the two previous case studies for good reason. According to 2017 data, an estimated 7.2 million people are living with HIV in South Africa, and it is estimated that the HIV prevalence rate for women aged 15–49 is 21.17 per cent. The effects of the epidemic – now towards the end of its fourth decade – have devastated young families especially. HIV complicates everything. It is a major driver of livelihood insecurity. With the death or disability of economically productive adults, HIV and AIDS have destabilised and eroded the social networks that sustain the livelihoods of vulnerable households. The impact of HIV is moderated because South Africa has the largest ART programme in the world, with active treatment programmes reducing the viral load, improving survival and preventing transmission. Even so, continued transmission accounts for a 250 000 new infections and 100 000 AIDS-related deaths each year. HIV and AIDS have placed chronic financial burdens on poor households, associated with health costs – not of the drugs but due to days missed from work – and the costs of attending health clinics and ensuring adequate nutrition. But there are indirect costs, too, associated with the continued stigma surrounding the infection. Kinship ties and other social connections are often undermined when someone has HIV, resulting in the withdrawal of support from some members of the immediate, as well as extended, family. The extended family, even the household, ceases to be a 'safety net' able to provide sanctuary and support in this context, again raising questions of the role of the state, community networks and NGOs (non-governmental organisations) in mitigating these effects and sustaining the care and support for affected individuals and their family members. Moreover, as the epidemic has aged (the first death in South Africa was recorded in 1985), common chronic problems with health – including concurrent HIV and cardiometabolic disease (obesity, diabetes and cardiovascular disease) – likely limit what care many adults can provide to each other. Both care needs and care tasks therefore may be shared among prime-aged and older adults, grand- and great-grandchildren.

In the following case study (5.5), Lario Viljoen, Hanlie Myburgh and Lindsey Reynolds draw upon research with home-based care workers and family members of 14 households directly affected by HIV and AIDS communities across the Cape Metro and Cape Winelands Districts, in the Western Cape Province. With this focus, they examine the fragile linkages between households and broader kin networks, highlighting the challenges that these households face in adapting to and managing the economic and social impact of the epidemic. Focusing on a mother, Bettie, and her daughter, Elsie, the case study's authors describe how managing health and negotiating healthcare is often a family affair. Bettie plays an essential role in shaping her daughter's understandings and experiences of health, including her willingness to adhere to ART to avoid a decline in her health, and, concurrently, to manage epilepsy, for which she also needs regular medication. This is complicated by the stigma and protective silence around HIV, but their absence in association with epilepsy. Bettie is Elsie's primary supporter, clinic companion, social guardian and health interpreter. How they manage Elsie's epilepsy and HIV illustrates the ways that close familial support extends beyond conventional notions of care and 'adherence support' to interpret health and rationalise care in unexpected ways.

Case study 5.5

A family affair

Lario Viljoen, Hanlie Myburgh and Lindsey Reynolds on behalf of the HPTN 071 (PopART) team[2]

The Jacobs family resides in a small informal community in the Cape Winelands District of South Africa. The community, which we call S-Town, includes 24 homes, wedged between an industrial area, a larger informal settlement, and a somewhat more affluent neighbourhood. The homes are all constructed of corrugated-iron sheets, boards and loose pieces of building material, salvaged from the neighbouring industrial area. Residents spend most of their time outside their homes, sitting in the sun, drinking and socialising. Together they also sort out materials for recycling, as is common among residents of the community. Daily life here is very much a public affair, and the boundaries of families and households are not always clearly demarcated. In this space, the management of chronic illness is often a profoundly social process.

The Jacobs family – the recognised matriarch Bettie (47), her long-term partner Ben (53), and their three children Elsie (23), Xavier (18) and Jerome (12) – are part of the social landscape of S-Town. Along with Jake (43), Elsie's partner, they make up the central core of a fluid household.[3] At any time, from two to five others, including members of the extended family, acquaintances, and friends, also stay with the family. We came to know the family when they were recruited to join a qualitative cohort study nested within a large-scale HIV-prevention trial in April 2016.[4]

In an early encounter, Bettie informed us discreetly that her daughter Elsie 'has the virus'. For some months after, however, HIV was an unspoken topic, a secret we shared with Bettie. By contrast, Elsie's epilepsy diagnosis was spoken of openly. When we first met Elsie she told us without prompting and in great detail about her epilepsy diagnosis and proudly showed us her medication, explaining how she manages the condition with the help of her mother, her family, others in the household, and other community members. She made no mention of any other health issues. On subsequent visits – whether we were standing outside their shack, near a neighbour's place, or inside their home – Elsie spoke openly about her epilepsy, often fetching her medication for public display. It took more than six months for her to disclose her HIV status, pointing her finger at the printed word 'HIV' on a survey form we were administering.

Reflecting on the different moments of disclosure, we were struck by how carefully Elsie and her family managed these intimate matters in a social and physical space that made privacy quite difficult to maintain. Bettie made it clear that we could talk openly about her daughter's epilepsy within and outside the household, but her HIV status was a private matter. While the two chronic conditions are central to her family's functioning, Elsie's interpretation of her illnesses and her decisions around disclosure are distinct. Elsie's story reveals not only the shading of revelations but the 'dimensions of secrecy' (Squire 2015: S206) related to illness and accessing support.

Public affliction, communal support

On a visit to the family in March 2017, we encountered Elsie, Jake and Sylvie, a transient household member, in the open area beside the house. Elsie's face was noticeably bruised and scabbed. In response to our concerned looks, she explained that the wounds were 'just from the epileptic attack [seizure]' that she had had two weeks earlier when she had been cooking on an open fire. Elsie 'literally just fell on her face,' Sylvie chimed in, attesting that Elsie had had no alcohol and had looked healthy before the incident. 'Elsie should not be in the sun too long,' Jake interjected, 'or stand next to the fire because of her epilepsy.' After the seizure, they told us, the neighbours helped Sylvie carry Elsie into her room. Elsie bandaged and applied ointment to the burns. Following this exchange, Jake and Sylvie returned to their task of sorting recycling, and we continued to walk with Elsie towards their home. She wanted to show us her medication again, which she keeps on a table in the room she and Jake share with Sylvie and her boyfriend. The medication is easily accessible and visible to all.

Since her epilepsy diagnosis in 2010, Elsie has meticulously attended her appointments at the local government clinic with her mother every two to three months. The clinic is a three-minute walk from her home.[5] It is her right to receive her medication, she adamantly explained to us, even if she finishes her tablets before her next scheduled visit and needs an unplanned medication top-up. With her mother's help, Elsie adjusts her dosage according to her needs. On most days, Elsie takes two tablets in the morning and two at night. If she experiences light-headedness, she takes an extra two to four tablets, sometimes eight tablets instead of the prescribed two.

As we finished our conversation, Bettie was waiting to talk with us, and the conversation gravitated towards Elsie's health, a constant concern of hers. She acknowledged that Elsie is 'a big girl' capable of taking responsibility for managing her illness, but she also knew that Elsie still relied on her support in various ways. Bettie accompanies Elsie to the clinic, helps monitor her treatment dosage, and facilitates Elsie's adherence to treatment. On one occasion, when Elsie left her medication at home while travelling, Bettie travelled several hours by train to take

Elsie's treatment to her. Bettie acts as a health interpreter for Elsie, helping her to make sense of her illness and its origin. She considers epilepsy as a family illness, since Elsie's father also had epilepsy as a child. In Bettie's account, Elsie's epilepsy was brought on by severe stress after she was raped as a child while the family was living in another nearby informal settlement.

Elsie's care is shared by others in the household and community. Household members offer daily assistance and advice, such as reminding her to stay out of the sun and away from the fire. During her seizures, the neighbours know how to get her 'right again'. Elsie explains that if they did not know to put a spoon in her mouth, she could lose her tongue. In addition, Elsie uses her epilepsy as a social shield. While she often gets into arguments with friends while drinking, she explains that others are careful not to fight with her because of the risk of seizures. Community members in S-Town are aware of Elsie's epilepsy and she can depend on them for support.

Elsie thinks of her home more as a community of support than a physical place, as she explains: 'I don't mind staying here. There aren't germs here. I don't pick up any diseases in this place. The health [condition] is from my family that gave it to me. What I have didn't come from this one or that one, or someone who gave it to me.' Although this might ring true for her epilepsy diagnosis, we wondered whether she had contracted HIV in S-Town also – a condition she manages in a very different way.

Private ailment, intimate care

When Elsie finally began to talk with us about her HIV status, she offered several different explanations of her infection. Her first and preferred explanation was that she became infected through contact with the blood of a sickly man in the community while helping him with house chores. But she also considered whether it could have been from her sexual assault as a child, although she had tested negative following the assault. We wondered if Elsie was trying to convince herself as well as us, or if she wanted to test the plausibility of these stories. Bettie, by contrast, was much more certain of how Elsie contracted HIV and had known long before she tested: 'A mother knows,' she explained, stating that she had noticed changes in Elsie's behaviour that suggested to her something was not right. At the time Elsie was swearing a lot, was overly aggressive, and had started to drink more than usual. Bettie expanded: 'Elsie had a boyfriend that she wasn't open to me about. And then we tested her and she had the virus.'

Secrecy is a dominant theme in the narrative about Elsie's HIV status. While Elsie's diagnosis is kept secret, according to Bettie, HIV also entered their household through a hidden relationship. The multiple and layered nature of disclosure and the dimensions of secrecy are evident in the ways in which Elsie and Bettie carefully consider whom to inform of either her epilepsy or HIV infection, weighed against the potential benefits or risks of secrecy and disclosure to her health and social wellbeing. Disclosing her HIV status to her close family offers the benefit of social support, but disclosure to the extended household and wider community may lead to social exclusion. In contrast to her epilepsy, Elsie's HIV status is kept hidden from everyone save for a few close family members, although it was not always clear who knew. Bettie told us that Ben and Jake were the only other household members who knew, but later Elsie said that she had also shared her status with her brothers. Extended-household members, temporary or permanent, were not aware. Bettie explained that if Elsie's HIV status was shared more widely, it would spread quickly to others within the small community.

Elsie's HIV was also collectively managed in a less direct way than her epilepsy. Elsie's HIV was not managed by medication, but by carefully keeping her status secret and attending to her diet so that she 'looks healthy'. Despite the family's limited income and food supply, Bettie and others ensured that Elsie had access to healthy food and provided her with ongoing encouragement, while attributing their concern for Elsie's health and her preferential treatment to her epilepsy.

Newly introduced national HIV-treatment guidelines recommend that all people living with HIV should be given access to treatment (DoH 2016), but Elsie stated that she had not been offered HIV treatment. Elsie, with Bettie's help, has come to interpret her need to start HIV treatment in terms of her perceived level of illness. Bettie explained that Elsie is not sick enough to start treatment, and that she only has 20 per cent of the illness; treatment is for those with levels of 50 per cent. Elsie reiterated that her HIV is not 'deep' because she contracted the virus through a cut in her hand, and therefore she does not need treatment. Both Bettie and Elsie maintained that the staff at the clinic had explained Elsie's HIV in this manner, and neither were clear about CD4 levels and treatment eligibility. The secretive manner in which Elsie's HIV status is handled also shapes how Elsie and her close family manage her illness.

Access to care for chronic conditions is subject to more than the availability of treatment or the distance to local clinics, as individuals try to make sense of and negotiate the daily realities of living with one or more illnesses. Perceived stigmatising attitudes from health staff and fellow community members can be major barriers to service access, especially for those seeking HIV treatment (Nyblade et al. 2013). Receiving treatment at clinics is also frequently associated with concerns about inadvertent public disclosure, even simply by 'being seen' to attend the clinic (Treves-Kagan et al. 2016).

On a day-to-day basis, Elsie's life is shaped by her epilepsy diagnosis, including her ability to provide for herself and her family, her reproductive intentions, her daily routines, and her sense of identity and community. But Elsie has embraced her diagnosis, and relies on household and community support for it; public knowledge of her epilepsy also serves at times as a social safeguard and allows her to conceal her HIV status. HIV, in contrast, is invisible and unspoken, mediated privately within a smaller, family sphere.

While epilepsy evidently marks Elsie's everyday social experience and self-management, on a national level, HIV disease has a greater tangible economic and social impact. In a high-burden country such as South Africa, where approximately 7.7 million people (or 13 per cent of the population) are living with HIV (UNAIDS 2016), the illness has become the country's chief public-health concern, and its management a matter for public intervention. Public-health stakeholders and implementers emphasise the importance of disclosure and treatment adherence to manage the illness and prevent transmission (see also Hodes, Vale and Toska's case study 5.3). These efforts occur alongside the increased decentralisation of HIV services into other community spaces and people's homes, bringing public management of the illness into the private domain. Yet Elsie's narrative illustrates how HIV is intimately managed and how it is instrumental for her and her family to keep it so. Conversely, epilepsy is also within the ambit of public health and is an often highly stigmatised disease, but Elsie manages it publicly and with community support.

Despite dominant narratives about the 'normalisation' of HIV and reductions in stigma (Persson 2013), many people still keep their diagnosis secret and make strategic choices about the elements of their illness experience they share with members of their families, households and communities (Adeniyi et al. 2017; George & McGrath 2019; Ramlagan et al. 2018). Understanding the intricate dynamics of how diseases are managed by individuals, households and communities can inform how health implementers interact with and assist individuals affected by co-morbidities.

South Africa has the highest number of people living with HIV in the world, and a high level of transmission of TB associated with HIV, with substance misuse, and with poor living conditions. But in addition, non-communicable diseases are among the leading causes of death in South Africa. Obesity and associated morbidities are increasing rapidly, where poor access to healthcare, limited economic resources, food insecurity and under-nutrition present formidable challenges. The contributing factors to both communicable and non-communicable diseases are therefore largely social.

In both urban and rural areas of South Africa, non-communicable chronic health problems – such as diabetes, asthma, cardiovascular disease and cancer – account for 20 per cent of mortality. These conditions – like all health and illness – are managed firstly within households. Although acute care may be needed at times – such as hospitalisation after a stroke – day-to-day care is home-based, undertaken by others close to those needing care; many of these caregivers also have chronic health problems. We have already noted that care is largely provided by householders, often reciprocally, and that it may also be provided by non-resident neighbours, family members and friends. Although grants may be provided to people to assist with caregiving under certain circumstances, formal non-acute care is limited. Government programmes for chronic medication – for instance, for diabetes and hypertension and HIV – including formal home- and facility-based care, are rare in both the public and private sectors, access is limited, and quality of care varies.

Cardiometabolic disease is precipitated and exacerbated by a range of social conditions, and biological factors interact and produce syndemics (Mendenhall & Norris 2015; Singer 2009; Singer et al. 2017). These interactions compound the effects of both biological and social factors, with each point of social vulnerability and/or physical health problem complicating others, resulting in a cascade of health problems at an individual level (Manderson & Warren 2016), and interpersonal and economic pressures within households and among families. For physiological and psychological reasons, depression is a co-morbidity of these various physical health problems, and its self-management (or lack of self-management) often leads to the misuse of alcohol and other drugs, with further implications in relation to health and wellbeing for individuals and family members.

Certain non-communicable conditions are particularly pernicious, and life threatening in the absence of early intervention. Without effective screening, diagnosis and treatment, cancer can be fatal, and fear of death often inhibits diagnosis and treatment-seeking at the outset (Mathews et al. 2015). South Africa has always been a place of contrasts, and those who have access to care and good treatment can expect to do well. Transplantation medicine shifts the experience of illness within households and among families, although again in complicated ways. With a kidney transplant, for instance, the temporality of daily life changes; the use of home space may change; and so may diet. Medication costs soar as immunosuppressant medication displaces the need for dialysis, often further impacting family welfare.

But other family-related issues influence decisions about whether or not to seek (and perhaps pay for) a transplant, about whether the organ is donated by a family member, and about testing to see whether the volunteer family member is compatible by blood type and tissue (Manderson 2011; Sharp 2006). The decision-making around the affordability and feasibility of a transplant places considerable stress on family members. Other modes of care that involve intimate bodily negotiations within families can also be fraught.

In the following case study (5.6), Emily Avera illustrates how the pursuit of bone-marrow stem-cell transplantation impacts family relationships. Drawing on field research conducted in 2015 and 2016 in Gauteng and Western Cape provinces, she describes how people diagnosed with leukaemia, lymphoma and other haematological disorders may be advised to have a bone-marrow stem-cell transplant provided that they can identify a related donor match. This shifts the relationships of patient and potential donors, and not always positively. In describing this, Alvera considers donors' experiences, and those of the health professionals who facilitate testing for compatibility and arrangements for treatment, swinging the analytic lens away from the family and back to the clinic, but with a keen eye on how medicalisation reshapes the family.

Case study 5.6

Blood ties

Emily Avera

Cary's principled steadfastness was one of the first things I noticed. A middle-aged man from a coloured community in Germiston in Gauteng Province, Cary (pseudonym) was the kind of person who prided himself on staying healthy, declaring he was drug and alcohol free. I interviewed him at the hospital where he had donated bone marrow (haematopoeitic) stem cells for a transplant to his sister. It was a private hospital with one of the largest bone-marrow stem-cell transplant units in South Africa.

In a gravelly voice, Cary described himself as a pillar of the community, an upstanding citizen in both body and mind. For 45 years he has ridden regularly on his bike around his neighbourhood as a postal delivery worker, and he told me, 'Nothing's wrong with my body because I've been active all the time.' Much of what he said suggested an unflappable countenance, physical strength, and certainty about his donation. However, he relayed a less sanguine, parallel narrative about the present state of his health and his perceptions about healthcare in South Africa. His whole life, he had relied on public healthcare. However, since his sister was on private medical aid and in need of a transplant, all aspects of the procedure were handled through the private healthcare system. The coverage included the entirety of Cary's donation process, from initial health screening, to donor–recipient cross-matching, to post-transplant checkups. This was his most extensive encounter with the private healthcare system. Cary's ruminations on the gaps between private and public healthcare were one of the most salient aspects of our conversation.

Cary conveyed his sense that the state of public healthcare in South Africa was troubled by corrupt mismanagement: 'Our public hospitals [have] great problems … most of the guys that should facilitate people with a lot of things, they'd rather steal the money. Some of them are even stealing the medicine to sell it.' From news headlines about the theft of medicines to personal experiences, he perceived stark differences between public healthcare and private healthcare. Cary saw varying levels of awareness and expertise between private and public doctors, partly from the specialisation of the private hospital transplant unit, but partly also from his sense of whether or not the clinicians understood or had resources to address his various health conditions, and how they might relate to what he underwent as a donor.

Cary's health concerns, he felt, were instigated or exacerbated by the donation. His prostate had swollen, and he required a catheter to urinate; he attributed this to the anaesthetic administered during the procedure. His arthritis was bad, and he recounted sometimes needing to stay at home in bed with severe pain. Even so, he reiterated never having health problems requiring an operation and being constantly active, while also conceding that perhaps his body could use a 'cool down' from incessant activity. While most other donors I spoke with had no post-transplant ailments, Cary's complaints raised questions about the reporting and tracking of donor health and safety (for overviews of the health of stem-cell donors, see Miller et al. 2008; Szer et al. 2016).

Cary's experiences illustrate the divide between public and private healthcare in South Africa. This gap can exist within families whose members have differential access to care (Mayosi & Benatar 2014). While not an attitude we should assume from a familial donor, Cary expressed a sense of moral clarity in donating to his sister and, like many other donors and advocates, he reasoned, 'What if it was you who needed help?' The contrast between him and his sister, whose medical-insurance cover enabled her to access excellent private treatment, and his critiques of public healthcare, indicated that this rationale and sense of familial obligation helped him balance any resentment of the transplant aftermath or the differential healthcare resources between siblings. Cary also had a concerned son living with him, and enjoyed a support system of friends and neighbours who helped him during the donation process and his bouts with illness.

Differences in public and private healthcare are often key to patients' experiences. However, the specificity of transplant patients' dependence on donors' merits deeper attention to donor perspectives and their social support. Experiences are partly contingent on financial means and health cover, but the clinical outcomes also hinge on family capacity to mobilise their kinship and community networks to fill gaps in care. Clinical outcomes are tied to family relationships in ways that health coverage cannot always account for.

Relational challenges

The costs of a transplant in relation to the other costs of clinical care may be straightforward when a compatible family donor is available and willing, but approximately 70 per cent of patients who need bone-marrow transplants cannot find family matches. Their next-best option is to search the South African Bone Marrow Registry (SABMR) for an anonymous, unrelated donor.[6] Donors are recruited and registered through the Sunflower Fund, an organisation founded by the mother of a patient who passed away and whose story led to the registration of hundreds of donors through community lobbying and to later several thousand more.[7] Although the goal is registering unrelated donors, the growth of the SABMR also illustrates how familial bonds indirectly impact patients' options.

Even when a willing related donor, adequate medical coverage and paid leave from employers are available, tensions in family relationships may develop or be exacerbated through the transplant process, and these can extend beyond the donor and recipient. For example, a woman named Lily donated to her youngest daughter, Kayla, who was suffering from lymphoma. She had no hesitation in caring for her daughter and donating stem cells to her, but Lily was troubled by the dynamics of her other family members. Lily had lost her husband earlier that year to poor health from his work in the mines, the primary source of economic opportunity in their home town. His recent death was a blow to their family, perhaps especially Kayla. Along with Kayla, Lily felt 'heartsore', a word she used as an English approximation for the Afrikaans sentiment of being *hartseer*. Kayla's sisters, although they were both healthy, were jealous and accused Lily of favouring Kayla. Lily was distressed by her other daughters' attitudes while she was trying to take care of her 'baby'. She struggled to make sense of their envy, juxtaposed with her own sense of duty: 'Why would I not take care of my child?'

Kayla's sisters were not viable donors. Had they been compatible, they would have been a clinically better option, since siblings are closer immunological matches than parents. Lily's donation fell into the haploidentical category of transplants – that is, a match with only half of the immunological types inherited from one parent. Only recently had the transplant unit begun to use this procedure in select cases, and clinicians regarded haploidentical transplants from parent to child as less effective clinical outcomes for the patient than transplants from sibling donors.[8] The procedure is one instance in which types of genetic kinship actually may affect treatment efficacy.

Foreclosures and futures

Nurses and social workers had a different perspective. They closely observe varied familial dynamics, donors, and patients, and their longer-term comprehension of the procedure provides insight into the challenges that families may face after the transplant. The lengthy aftermath of a successful transplant can be a struggle for patients, donors and other family members, especially if they perceive a transplant to be curative and definitive rather than requiring constant management. Social workers and bone-marrow-transplant advocates who had close relationships with patients and families spoke in grave tones of those who, following a successful transplant, experienced problems with other issues. For example, they were unable to maintain proper recovery conditions (such as providing access to good sanitation facilities, or ensuring restricted contact with people outside the home), or they were unprepared for the feelings of isolation that immunologically vulnerable patients experience when they must stay at home to convalesce and avoid potentially fatal infections. Familial relationships were often strained; for example, marriages floundered due to the effects of transplant treatments on patients' sexual function. For every patient featured in publicity material running marathons after a transplant, others relapse, suffer from depression, or develop physical limitations. Sometimes families face financial and emotional hardships due to the high costs of the pre-transplant treatment, the transplant itself, and the immunosuppressant regimen thereafter (Manderson 2011; Sharp 2006).

During my time in the haematology unit, the doctors, the nurses and the social worker shared recollections of patient and related-donor tensions, which threatened to foreclose any possibility of a related transplant. Unit staff preferred patients to approach their relatives to get tested and about their willingness to donate. Only then would the donor connect with hospital staff. However, familial ties and obligations did not always result in moral clarity for potential donors, and public-hospital staff often intervened. Relatives' reluctance or refusal can stem from 'bad blood' superseding blood-bound notions of familial care. Conflicts were insurmountable at times, as one hospital worker explained:

> We had a case … a young girl … she had leukaemia, but we refused to
> treat her unless she had a sibling donor. Her siblings weren't a match, but
> her mother and her mother's sister married two brothers, so there was
> actually a chance of the first cousins being perfect matches. There was
> some family dispute between the two families and the cousins actually
> refused to come even though she was terminally ill. She had leukaemia
> and she died and they had no remorse. And there was a good chance that
> … she actually could have been saved. And she was young, she was about
> 19 or 20. Very difficult, family disputes … the doctors tried to intervene,
> the social workers, you name it, we got involved.

Sometimes tensions arise because donors do not realise that they may have to return after their initial donation. If the initial harvest of stem cells is sufficient, it can be disorienting to be asked to return to provide an additional donation, so straining the relationship between related donors and recipients. One nurse recounted:

> We had a patient here, Mr Bertram, and his donor was very upset because
> she had to donate twice, and she had to stay out of work and go through
> all the trauma financially too, and emotionally, and she got no satisfaction
> out of it. She didn't actually want to donate.

Another nurse recalled:

> The relationship [was] not good between the donor and the patient. This
> was the second time with her as well … and he even threatened the donor,
> [saying], 'If you don't go and do the bone marrow and donate, then I am
> going to take you the police.' She was just doing a favour for him, and
> now he was threatening her and she didn't know that if she doesn't donate
> there won't be anything that will happen to her. She was just thinking,

'Okay, if I don't donate then I will be in trouble.' [The patient] he owns a taxi, and apparently this was taken by the donor's husband so [the patient] was claiming some money from them … I spoke to the donor and she also phoned the husband so they were prepared to give back all the money that they were owing him.

The repeated need for donation was a point of contention in each of these stories. Finances and property were pivotal, and patients occasionally used threats as a stratagem to compel donation. In the public hospital, which serves a wide cross-section of races and socioeconomic classes, the clinicians pointed out to me that these cases of strife were all in 'lower-income' families. These recollections contrasted sharply with stories of donation in private hospitals, which were not marked by coercion. Staff experience with 'middle- to high-income' patients and donors was completely different. They told me of how a patient could afford the fee to search the Australian bone-marrow registry to find a matching donor not related by familial ties: 'The day the [potential match] heard we were looking for a donor, he jumped on the next plane and came for tissue typing. Just flew for tissue typing and he was a match. And for the transplant, he also flew in at his own expense.'

At the private transplant unit, among high-income patients, nurses witnessed a trend of families who would go to extreme financial lengths, hoping to enhance patient care, with desperation leading them to push for treatment measures with little efficacy but hefty expense. Families were more at loggerheads about escalating expenditures than engaging in compensatory disputes, as seen in the public hospital with low-income families. These cases demonstrate the different dilemmas between those who bear the burden as a large percentage of their income or risk financial ruin, and those who do not. Nurses witnessed middle- and high-income families expend resources to exhaust every option. Families who found themselves in debt post-transplant often harboured resentment toward the patient. Regardless of patient outcome, high costs and debt could seriously jeopardise families' financial futures, even drastically shifting their socioeconomic position.

For relatively costly donor-dependent medical procedures such as transplantation, the divide between public and private healthcare produces stark differences in lived experiences. Access to treatment and optimisation of clinical outcomes may depend both on specific genetically material relationships between family members, and on the social character of the relationships. In some cases, the search for a match tests the limits of these kin relationships biomedically, socially and financially. In other cases, the importance of family is reaffirmed, or the differences and conflicts are thrown into relief.

Family-based care includes the everyday care delivered within households, where health is an outcome of access to sufficient potable water, hygiene and sanitation, food and shelter. In other words, caregiving is synonymous with the household; being part of a household implies the capacity and willingness to provide and receive care in some respects. But, as has been illustrated, the preconditions for good enough care are absent in many South African households, and so the capacity to care and the quality of care are compromised. The state supports people in the most precarious positions, but to a limited degree. While grants, institutional care and free services are critical, these may be insufficient to ensure the wellbeing of household members.

In the case studies included in this chapter, we have focused on a range of issues that connect individuals, households, families and services: how communities support the parents of young and middle-aged children, and how parents manage their immediate environments to protect their family in toxic settings. We have considered how parents struggle with their own health problems and those of their children, including, as may be expected, of HIV infection. While these may be issues of the present, family capacity to respond is a constant reminder of South Africa racist legacy. We have, in addition, explored the family cooperation required to manage co-morbidity – and any health problem – and the challenges for family members when asked to step into the medicalised role of donor.

Notes

1   Street pesticides are much less expensive than other consumer products designed for domestic use on pests, but are also much more hazardous, and therefore more effective in killing unwanted pests.

2   Special thanks to the Jacobs family and the HPTN 071 (PopART) study team and sponsors for the opportunity to contribute to this publication. The HPTN 071 study is sponsored by the National Institutes of Health (NIH), the medical research agency of the USA. Primary funding is from the National Institute of Allergy and Infectious Diseases (NIAID) under Cooperative Agreements UM1-AI068619, UM1-AI068617, and UM1-AI068613, with funding from the US President's Emergency Plan for AIDS Relief (PEPFAR). Additional funding is provided by the International Initiative for Impact Evaluation (3ie) with support from the Bill & Melinda Gates Foundation, as well as by NIAID, the National Institute on Drug Abuse (NIDA) and the National Institute of Mental Health (NIMH), all part of NIH. The content is solely the responsibility of the authors and does not necessarily represent the official views of the NIAID, NIMH, NIDA, PEPFAR, 3ie, or the Bill & Melinda Gates Foundation.

3   In this account, we use the terms 'household' and 'family' in quite specific ways. Cognisant of the broader debate within the literature on the difference between these terms and the boundaries of collective social forms (Reynolds 2015), we employ the two terms to draw out an important distinction our interlocutors made between the different layers of intimacy and relatedness within their home. The term 'household' is used to refer to the fluid social grouping that resides together in their home. This household can be formed and reformed to accommodate acquaintances, friends, and relatives in times of need. The Jacobs 'family', by contrast, is understood to be a relatively stable 'nuclear' unit.

4   The larger trial within which this cohort study was nested – HPTN 071 (PopART) – is a cluster-randomised trial of an HIV-prevention strategy often referred to as 'universal test and treat' (UTT). The Jacobs family lives in one of the control arms of the trial. They were not exposed to the trial intervention. For more details on the overall trial structure, see Hayes et al. (2014).

5   In South Africa, the national Department of Health has attempted to ensure that all South Africans have access to affordable and geographically obtainable basic healthcare through an estimated 4 200 local community clinics and state-run hospitals (Makombo 2016). Despite concerns about quality of care, for most South African citizens, the government-run clinics are the primary source of medical treatment, including antenatal care, mental-health support, immunisations, and treatment and support for chronic conditions such as TB, epilepsy, high blood pressure, diabetes and HIV (DoH 2017; Makombo 2016).

6   A local registry search does not guarantee that a matching donor is available. Patients with the means (or through fundraising) will extend their search to registries in other countries. Generally, none of the added costs of overseas donations – including a courier who must cross international borders to procure the stem cells for transplantation – are covered by medical aids in South Africa. Despite such efforts, patients can still fail to find matches. The feasibility of a transplant varies according to financial means, but it is also affected by varying probabilities of finding a compatible donor on registries (for more on matching and donor recruitment, see Avera 2009).

7   Much could be said about the role of kinship networks in many donor-recruitment organisations worldwide. Like the Sunflower Fund, these are often founded by friends and family when a related donor is unavailable and they begin large-scale public campaigns to find donors.

8   While clinical outcomes for haploidenticals can be equivalent to other transplants (Di Stasi et al. 2014), at the time of fieldwork the predominant perspective of clinicians with whom I spoke was that this was less effective.

6 *As families age*

Lenore Manderson and Nolwazi Mkhwanazi

Life expectancy in South Africa is comparatively low as a result of HIV prevalence and structural inequalities. Still, by 2017, in the absence of HIV infection, men could expect to live to 64.5 years and women 71.5 years, in contrast to life-expectancy rates in 2002 of 61.4 for men and 68.3 for women (Stats SA 2018). Estimates of life expectancy that include HIV infection are both more realistic and depressing: 48.7 years for men and 50.7 years for women in 2015 (He et al. 2016: 34).

Even so, with improved treatments that enable people to live for an extended period with chronic communicable diseases – including HIV and TB – and non-communicable conditions such as cardiometabolic (diabetes and cardiovascular) diseases, South Africa is ageing rapidly. Increased longevity comes at a price, with increasing co-morbidities and complications, and other concurrent conditions. An older person might, for instance, have diabetes, with retinopathy and peripheral neuropathy, and heart disease, depression, and perhaps vascular dementia associated with the primary condition. Unrelated, they may also have arthritis and chronic obstructive pulmonary disease. This person therefore may face challenges relating to controlling their underlying symptoms (such as high blood glucose and hypertension), stabilising the conditions, ensuring adequate and appropriate diet and nutrition, controlling pain, managing mobility and self-care, meeting the costs of attending clinics for monitoring and adjustment of treatments, and meeting the costs of some pharmaceuticals. HIV infection and adherence to ARVs (antiretrovirals) adds to this complexity.

With the accumulation of health problems, there is an increasing need for active caregiving. This might be limited to checking adherence to medication, but might also include taking on various domestic tasks and – depending on the capacity of the individual – assisting with bathing, cooking, dressing and other self-care. Changes in household size and composition mean that this is not always straightforward. In earlier chapters, we noted that there are fewer formal marriages and that women are having fewer children. These trends and more deaths and outmigration are leading to smaller households (Collinson et al. 2007), and high levels of migration for work (Camlin et al. 2013). High rates of divorce, unofficial cohabitation, single parenthood and other kinds of living arrangements work against strong norms to care for others, including elders. The fragility of households and families impacts on the availability and provision of care and support. Often, too, people who might be seen as caregivers may also have chronic health problems, pre-existing and acquired over time, and may struggle to care for themselves and others. The severity of the health condition(s) of householders, including fluctuations in mobility, capacity, physical-health status and frailty, impacts on care needs. People 60 years and older are entitled to receive a grant – the Older Person's Grant – subject to a means test, and this is at times the main or sole source of household income. Further, in both rural and urban South Africa many factors influence the size and strength of social and kin networks, and the willingness and ability of others in these networks to provide additional economic, physical and emotional support.

There is limited formal non-acute care in South Africa coordinated by government or NGOs (non-governmental organisations). There are few affordable residential-care homes, few day-care programmes, and limited support provided by primary healthcare workers and community volunteers (Nxumalo et al. 2016). Care for people who are aged, frail and living with a number of diseases and debilitating conditions falls on householders or non-resident neighbouring kin and non-kin. Many people, including ageing couples, try to care for themselves and each other in extreme poverty and with limited resources of all types, even basic working infrastructure such as taps (Nxumalo et al. 2016).

In case study 6.1, Monde Makiwane, Ntombizonke A Gumede and Mzolisi Makiwane consider the challenges faced by elderly people in South Africa. Based on research conducted in a resource-poor rural environment near Mthatha in the Eastern Cape province, the authors describe the life of Tsogo, an 84-year-old man without formal education. Drawing on global and national discourse (HSRC 2012; WHO 2017) around 'healthy ageing', Makiwane, Gumede and Makiwane trace the strategies Tsogo used, which he believes have contributed to living a healthy and active life. In this context, they illustrate the value of intergenerational solidarity, social connection, and active life, as well as access to nutritious foods to maximise health.

Case study 6.1

Healthy ageing

Monde Makiwane, Ntombizonke A Gumede and Mzolisi Makiwane

Tsogo is 84 years old, and yet he seems much younger. He is still employed as a heavy-duty truck driver, and sometimes undertakes long return trips of more than 3 000 kilometres. He shows no signs of slowing down. Many turn their heads when his age is mentioned, shaking their heads in disbelief.

According to the WHO (World Health Organization), 'healthy ageing' should be defined as the 'development and maintenance of optimal mental, social and physical well-being and function in older adults'. When we write of healthy ageing, we are referring to the postponement of or reduction in the undesired effects of ageing. The goals include maintaining physical and mental health, avoiding disorders, and remaining active and independent. However, ageing in Africa occurs against a background of socioeconomic hardship. Most older people live in rural areas where there is often very little access to basic services and markets. While family ties remain strong, traditional support systems have changed. The migration of younger adults and the impact of HIV and AIDS have led to a rise in the number of skip-generation households, consisting of older people (often a grandparent) and children.

South Africa is country of glaring contrasts: a developing world with an upper-middle-income economy; a sea of poverty in rural areas; and the periphery of urban centres characterised by sprawling informal settlements on the margins of evergreen golf estates and posh suburbs displaying vast urban wealth. Life expectancy is one aspect of South African life that clearly reflects these contrasts.

Being elderly is characterised by high levels of functional difficulty, such as struggling to walk and having poor sight and hearing. Thrown into this mix, gender, race and class interact to shape the everyday experiences, and development and health outcomes, of older persons in South Africa (Makiwane et al. 2012). This is related to historical disadvantage of certain groups in South Africa, particularly the majority African population. Women are more likely to belong to the lowest socioeconomic class, but they are in a better state of health and live longer than men. Older African men have the worst health status of all.

Tsogo is an exception. His story sharply contrasts with the main narrative of ageing in South Africa, and suggests the value of investigating African men from low socioeconomic backgrounds who are ageing healthily. Tsogo leads a very simple life, which still pays allegiance to African value systems and ways of life, yet he has successfully negotiated contemporary life. Other men and women too, from a similar background, seem to be outliers from the statistical norm. This poses a question of what social factors, not captured by current longevity studies, contribute to longevity.

The early years

Tsogo was born into a family of farm workers, one of six children – he is the only one still living. His parents worked for a farm owner throughout their adult life, although they changed employers when the first farm they worked on was sold. The new farm owners and employers were unlike many other farmers, who ill-treated their workers. Tsogo's father owned his own cattle and sheep; his parents tilled their own land and grew maize and vegetables. Tsogo took on chores at an early age, herding calves and then family stock. He hunted animals, ate wild berries and nuts, played at stick fights, swam, went to youth evening party events (*imitshotsho*), and, like most Xhosa boys of his time, underwent *ukwaluka* (circumcision) as essential to the transition to adulthood. He was taught that to be a man was to be responsible. Tsogo started working as a labourer on the farm on which he had grown up. His early farming duties revolved around cattle herding. At the same time, he started his own farming and stock-rearing, at which he became adept. He grew his stock to a herd of 25 cattle and 50 sheep.

Tsogo, as taught by his father, valued and nurtured relationships. He developed a good relationship with his employer, a white middle-class man, and his employer's family; and their relationship remains strong to this day, marked by frequent telephone calls between the families and invitations to each other's important family events. This relationship extends to the wider family. Tsogo often spends time with the farmer's daughter over a cup of tea whenever he is in East London.

When Tsogo was young, men dreamt of leaving their farms and moving to the city of gold, Johannesburg, in search for wealth and adventure. When Tsogo made this journey, he nearly did not reach the city. On his way, he was intercepted by police forced by the apartheid government to limit and control the movements of African people into urban areas. Tsogo's good relations with his farm bosses saved him. They assured the police that he was going to the city for a short period and that he would not abandon rural life – he was a successful farmer who owned a lot of stock. The police were persuaded, and Tsogo was able to proceed to Johannesburg.

Social connections

Tsogo's life has been enriched by social capital. He values social interactions and communication. He spends a lot of time connecting with relatives on a cellphone – spending about R200 a day speaking to relatives, near and far, using a daily personal allowance from his employers, airtime from children and rebates from the cellphone company. He routinely makes calls to children, grandchildren, in-laws, and others in the extended family. Intergenerational solidarity was ingrained by Tsogo's parents, who emphasised family priority and held family in higher esteem than individual members. Cellphone technology has made social connection a reality among members of different generations that are geographically dispersed. Tsogo's social connections, moreover, are not confined to family; a man of faith, he interacts regularly with church members. When available, he is often asked to preach in church and regularly attends community meetings; in deference to his age, he is often given a ceremonial role at these. TM Nhongo (2004) explains that in most African societies older persons remain relevant in society by being made family and community counsellors, and given ceremonial roles in society.

At home Tsogo is a story teller of note. He grew up in a household in which, in the evenings, family members gathered together in the children's hut for stories of different kinds. This was a home theatre, Tsogo explains, where people would wind down in preparation for a night's sleep. Tsogo relives his childhood memories as he retells these stories to his own children and grandchildren. On these nights he becomes animated, as the family sits to listen to him and he mimics the sounds of birds, wild and domesticated. He relates his childhood hobbies, his childhood home and experiences. He tells the story of the mischief of the *imbila* (dassie) during their hare-hunting episodes as boys. Hares keep to mountainous areas although they also skirt the foot of the mountain in search for food. They scurry up mountains to escape hunting teams, and once at a safe distance, they become mischievous and turn to mock the hunters. When Tsogo tells such stories he becomes animated, acts them out, imitating the *imbila*, the roosters, and the various animals he is narrating. Children and other listeners respond with warm, roaring laughter and giggles. These stories continue the old African tradition of entertaining, informing, transmitting values, passing on history to the younger generations. They also help to foster strong bonds of family relations.

Education

Neither Tsogo nor his siblings attended school, despite the fact that there was a farm school and the farm owners encouraged schooling. His father was against his children going to school, concerned that schooling would influence children to abandon their cultural and societal values, and to lose their humanity and manhood or womanhood. Long distances to the farm school and lack of transport further mitigated against formal education.

In Johannesburg, Tsogo worked as an underground miner. He was focused and productive, and was quickly promoted to a supervisory position. Parallel to working, he attended a mine night-school for literacy, but, unhappy with his supervisory position, he decided to leave mining and move back to the farm. However, his return to the farm was short lived. Tsogo had tasted the advantages of town life, especially of education, and resolved that his children would get formal education. Tsogo moved to Cala, a nearby village, with his family, and worked as a driver for a hotel establishment. Later he worked in Cape Town, then moved to Mthatha, where he and his family now reside. He still works as a truck driver.

Employment

A priority area in the South African *Plan of Action on Ageing* (DoSD 2002) and the African Union *Policy Framework and Plan of Action on Ageing* (AU 2003) is the inclusion of older people as active participants in the labour force. Older persons are among the most vulnerable, and there have been suggestions that the age of retirement – currently, in most occupations, either 60 or 65 years – should be raised. Debates on retirement have been prompted by the global increase of the aging population, especially in high-income settings such as Japan and Italy, where the population of people 65 years and older is 33.4 per cent and 29.4 per cent respectively (UN 2017). In South Africa, concern also relates to the precarious living conditions of older people. Most South Africans, irrespective of race, are financially ill prepared for old age.

Tsogo is currently employed as a truck driver and is still lively. He usually leaves home just after 6 a.m., sometimes earlier, and returns at about 7 p.m. In the two days preceding our interview with him, he had risen at 3 a.m. on two consecutive cold winter days and returned at about 7 p.m. each night, spending most of these days driving and supervising assistants loading and offloading the truck. Most trips are a couple of hundred kilometres long, but some are further – he routinely travels over 1 000 kilometres from Mthatha to Cape Town. His company offered him a co-driver, but he refused, preferring lone driving to avoid the long breaks on the way that others might request. His routine work week is six days; if needed, he works for seven days.

Tsogo challenges the assumptions about old people as consumers and dependents, reliant on pension funds, other public transfers and family care. In South Africa, the government has been looking at ways of linking old-age pensions to self-employment (Zuma 2017). While steps have been taken to enforce this, research and policy responses lack ways to strengthen the economic security of older people, and there is limited information on elderly participation in the labour force and the circumstances under which it is available.

Research by Metropolitan found that 40 per cent of people have no form of retirement savings (Old Mutual 2017). Other insurance and life-assurance companies consistently draw attention to the limited number of people in formal employment, and especially in the informal sector, who have pension arrangements, and associate this with low financial literacy (see, for example, Sanlam Wealthsmiths 2016). Further, although a proportion of people have retirement funds, their contributions are insufficient to sustain their lifestyles, and although the old-age non-contributory pension scheme is well established, it is often inadequate. This is particularly so when older people support younger family members in the context of high unemployment and increased numbers of orphaned children.

Diet

Tsogo's diet is typical of traditional Xhosa societies. He usually eats two full meals a day, in the middle of the day and in the evening. Both meals consist of samp (partly ground corn, the most popular staple food among amaXhosa) and *amasi* (fermented milk). His meals are usually accompanied by fresh vegetables, cultivated by his wife in their garden. When time permits, Tsogo also works in the garden, and his wife maintains that he has a 'green thumb' when planting pumpkins. His gardening includes mending fences and fixing garden tools, and this physical activity is an important component of his health. Tsogo's philosophy of food is simple: eat in moderation, avoid fatty foods, and eat fresh food as often as possible.

Health status

Tsogo is full of vitality, brimming with health and young looking; he rarely suffers ailments, except occasionally flu. As far as he can remember, he has had one operation, related to a urological problem. He visits a family doctor on a regular basis for health check. This is consistent with traditional norm. AmaXhosa had family doctors and priests, *amagqirha* (diviners). Christian families continue that trend by visiting traditional doctors. The family doctor who regularly examines Tsogo confirms he has none of the common non-communicable diseases associated with ageing. His blood pressure and other common health indicators of ageing are comparable to a healthy person who has not reached their sixties. His medical doctor thinks that one of Tsogo's remarkable traits is his ability to remain calm; as an example, the doctor referred to the occasion when Tsogo tragically lost a son to a car accident, yet he remained serenely peaceful and calm. Absence of anxiety is one source of his good life, his doctor explains. Xhosa men are groomed to be the pillars of strength during storms. Calmness is a hallmark of Xhosa manhood. Men are stabilisers and absorbers of shocks in the family. The ability to appear calm is a quality of cultural and traditional notions of manhood among amaXhosa, supported by social structures and encouraged in men assuming the roles of strategic thinkers and protectors.

Unemployment levels are high in rural South Africa. Those who are able take advantage of employment opportunities when they can, finding work locally as labourers on infrastructure projects, on farms, on game reserves and in services, or as waged workers in the commercial agricultural sector. Women working on farms in commercial agriculture are paid less than men and are less likely than men to receive formal work contracts, and are more often informally employed, with little job protection or security (Devereux 2019). The vulnerability to which women are subject as workers influences their ability to self-care and to care for other householders, on both a routine and an emergency basis. The implications are these: if the primary caregiver – however this is determined – is in paid employment, then those who need care may be left alone for extended periods of time; health-care appointments may be deferred if a caregiver needs to take time off work; and the health problems of the caregiver may be ignored. In addition, increasingly women rather than men migrate for work, returning only intermittently for family gatherings, at Christmas and Easter, and for emergencies. In consequence, fewer householders are available to take on the mundane and higher-need caregiving of co-resident grandchildren and other minors, frail older people, or others requiring assistance with everyday living. Often, as has already been noted, the caregivers are themselves elderly, and may need to provide high-level care while their own health is compromised or declining.

In the following case study (6.2), Lenore Manderson examines how the provision of care is managed in a rural village in Mpumalanga Province. The village of Nsimu consists of some 700 households and a population of about 4 000, and so it is relatively large, and it is divided into two administrative sections. It is situated in the Bushbuckridge Local Municipality, some 29 kilometres east of the municipal centre of Bushbuckridge and 41 kilometres south of the town of Acornhoek and Tintswalo Hospital, the only public hospital in the municipality. Nsimu is also 10 kilometres from Agincourt, from where the Rural Public Health and Health Transitions Research Unit (Agincourt Unit) operates (Kahn et al. 2012); it was through the auspices of the unit that Manderson and an assistant, Marcia Vilakazi, were introduced to community-health workers, village leaders and others. Drawing on interviews undertaken with elderly householders and care providers primarily in 2017, Manderson highlights the difficulties faced by people living in extremely poor circumstances with limited capacity to self-care, and reflects on the limits to local interventions to support them.

Case study 6.2

Caring, communities and poverty

Lenore Manderson

Disparities are vast in South Africa, by class, race and gender, and between urban and rural areas. In rural Mpumalanga Province, this plays out in the capacity of householders to provide care to both children and elders. For older frail people, the home environment can be particularly important in terms of general health and longevity (Makiwane et al. 2004), but as I discuss below, an optimal – even a good enough – environment is difficult in poor rural settings.

In Nsimu, cardiometabolic conditions (hypertension, stroke and diabetes) contribute significantly – along with the continued high prevalence of HIV and TB – to morbidity and mortality. This is also the case elsewhere in the municipality of Bushbuckridge, as documented in the past two decades (Bocquier et al. 2014; Clark, Gómez-Olivé et al. 2015; Gaziano et al. 2017; Gómez-Olivé et al. 2014). These conditions occur concurrently with a range of other disabling and degenerative conditions: vision loss; hearing loss; poor dental health; asthma and other respiratory problems; urinary incontinence; arthritis and related conditions impacting mobility; mild cognitive decline; depression; and – an emerging problem with increased longevity – Alzheimer's disease and other dementias. In addition, acute respiratory and gastrointestinal problems are common. For most of these conditions, people require some assistance from others for personal care and everyday household activity, in external interactions (shopping, banking and so on), and in presenting for medical care. Some people require more intensive care and assistance in core activities of daily living, including communication, dressing, bathing, toileting and feeding. Usually, as was indicated earlier in this chapter, none of these conditions occurs in isolation; instead, multiple conditions accrue and intensify with ageing. Poverty erodes household capacity to manage multiple conditions, and the greater the number, the greater the economic and personal burden: more trips to doctors, more medicines, more personal care, more expenses (Manderson & Warren 2016).

In Nsimu, over 50 per cent of people aged 15–60 are unemployed; with limited literacy and formal education, they have few opportunities. Those who are employed travel considerable distances for commercial farm-labouring jobs or employment in the service sector, such as on private game reserves. Because of these long distances, many choose to live closer to work. They neither contribute to the household practically nor earn enough to supplement household finances. Only one interviewee reported receiving regular financial support from his children and was relatively comfortable. However, older people contributed significantly to their households because they receive a government pension of R1 500 per month; if they were caring for grandchildren, they were entitled to the CSG (Child Support Grant). In theory, the pension is intended to meet their own living and medical costs; in practice, this was sometimes the only cash covering the costs of food, clothing, educational expenses, utilities and data for phones, as well as transport for shopping, healthcare and medication. Nurses and care workers reported that older people often had little control over the use of grant money, with relatives reportedly taking the money from them. Those who needed substantial assistance, and who lived alone or without other adults to aid them, sometimes tried to buy in help. This was not always easy. Vukosi, for example, paid a cleaner R500 to work for three days a week; the arrangement ended after three weeks when the cleaner demanded R600 a week. It was also not a viable option in the long term, since the cost of paid help was greater than Vukosi's grant.

Poverty was perceptible throughout Nsimu. People lived in houses they had often built themselves over an extended period of time; the area was dotted with small, half-built brick houses. In 11 of the 20 households with people over the age of 60 in which we conducted interviews, kitchen, bathing facilities and toilets (most often, unlined pit latrines) were located outside the house. Those who were not mobile depended on others to cook for them and take them to the toilet. Pipes leaked or were broken; the houses were damp; the floors were dirty; and there were problems with mould, dust and pests (see Levine, Swartz and Rother's case study 5.1). People frequently stored both food and water outside the house; furniture was sparse and sometimes broken. A resident, Ponani, reflected, 'With the storms of 2014, my house was destroyed. I have only been able to replace the windows. The house has holes and cracks; cockroaches and rats have taken over. I have no bed, no decent furniture. All my clothes have holes.'

Access to health services was problematic, because bus services were infrequent and many people who were elderly and frail were unable to travel alone. Although hospitals and major medical centres were located around an hour or so away by car, travel for people from Nsimu, and elsewhere in the district, took far longer. Kulani, another resident, explained:

> I have to ask an unemployed lady across the street to travel with me as I cannot travel alone. I leave early in the morning and take four taxis [minibus shared taxis] to get our destination at Bongani Hospital [41 kilometres south] for my monthly medical checkup, then travel four taxis back, paying for both of us each way.

Andzisa, a resident who can no longer walk, added to this: 'As you can see, my legs don't work. I have to drag myself to the main road to get a taxi, which drops me away from the clinic, then I drag myself to the centre. Once a month, every month, for my check up and medicine.'

Older people were often reluctant to seek care for other reasons: there were long waiting times; they could not always see the doctor; communication with providers was limited; diagnoses and treatment were not explained; they were afforded little privacy when they presented for care; and they felt disrespected. While others might say the same of quality of care in primary healthcare services elsewhere in Bushbuckridge and nationwide, participants believed that they were especially slighted because they were old.

Nurses, from their side, were concerned by patient delay, with people presenting only when desperately ill. Nurses affirmed how poverty influenced this: elderly people were reluctant to go to a medical centre because of lack of food and clean clothes. In an effort to improve access, the province had introduced mobile clinics to travel to villages on a weekly basis, but this was unreliable. The mobile clinic did not operate in November and December 2016, for instance. When the clinic resumed operating in 2017, clinic nurses resorted to filling expired scripts, using their own phones to call doctors at the hospital to check if they could do so for patients with chronic conditions whose health was deteriorating.

In response to the problems of poor healthcare and poverty, one of the churches in Nsimu decided to extend a programme that had been established to provide food and supervised homework sessions for children considered to be orphaned, destitute or neglected. Like other innovations in the region (see Jessica Ruthven's case study 6.5), the church was able to employ care workers through a grant from the Department of Social Development, to provide after-school meals for children and deliver food parcels to households. In doing so, the care workers identified frail elderly and chronically ill householders. These were often people whose children had migrated to cities for work, while they elected to stay in familiar surroundings. Using some of the funds intended for children, the care workers began to assist older people to bathe; they cooked, cleaned and washed clothes for them; and – for those who were sufficiently mobile to get to the church – they extended the church-based meals programme to them two days a week. The care workers had no skills, however, to meet the other needs of those they began to visit: to care for wounds, to advise on treating infections, or to help them manage incontinence and medication. Frustrated, the scheme was at risk of collapse, and older people had stopped coming to the church for meals. In January 2017, however, a group of volunteers began to operate out of an unused outside room, in poor condition, of a deceased estate. At the time of the research, soon after they moved in to this 'office', they were debating the range of activities that might be feasible.

Sustainability is a challenge for such initiatives: those supported by the government (such as the mobile clinics), and those initiated by community members (such as the home visits to the elderly). Although in some cases larger NGOs may step in to fund local activities, most home-visiting and day-care programmes are supported through funds from the Department of Social Welfare. These programmes are still rare, and they depend on the commitment of those who establish them. Under conditions of poverty and precariousness, characteristic of this area, any shift in the circumstances of the care workers, and their households and families, jeopardises their capacity to support others who are both vulnerable and frail.

In October 2015, the Department of Health of Gauteng Province terminated an outsourced care contract with a private healthcare provider, Life Esidimeni, as a measure to 'deinstitutionalise' psychiatric patients, although there were also cost savings to the province. From March to December 2016, an estimated 1 300 people were transferred to the care of their families, hospitals and NGOs, many of which lacked competence and experience in providing appropriate care and were poorly resourced (Freeman 2018; Van Rensburg et al. 2018). Subsequent inquiry drew attention to the horrendous circumstances of people's transfer and lack of care; 143 people died from – while others survived – personal neglect, starvation, lack of medical care and inappropriate medication. The Life Healthcare Esidimeni scandal highlighted then – as it still does – the lack of attention to mental-health problems in South Africa. The scandal drew attention to people who were already out of family care, living in institutions or on the streets.

Even so, the majority of people with mental-health problems – including those with anxiety, depression and substance-use problems, and with bipolar disorder and schizophrenia – live with families. Their health problems reverberate within the households in which they reside, with implications for the emotional wellbeing – and sometimes physical health – of others, and for the economic stability of the household as a unit. In the following case study (6.3), Stine Hellum Braathen and Leslie Swartz draw on data from Braathen's doctoral research conducted in rural Eastern Cape in 2012. They describe the care afforded to one older woman, Ntombali, with a severe mental disorder. Nomabali's immediate household, and an extended network of family members, ensure that she is cared for well; concurrently, members of the family work together to support others in the household too. This does not imply that caregiving is easy, and, as we see, care burden affects the entire household, immediate and extended. Nomabali's care, the authors illustrate, is constrained by household and community poverty and lack of health services, and this influences the wellbeing of all who are providing support.

Case study 6.3

Nomabali's story

Stine Hellum Braathen and Leslie Swartz

In Eastern Cape Province – one of the poorest, most highly populated and neglected provinces of South Africa – lies a deep rural area known as Madwaleni. The majority of people living here are amaXhosa people from the Bomvana clan. In 2012, while exploring care for people with mental disorders in Madwaleni, I (Stine) met Nomabali, a 77-year-old Xhosa woman. My interpreter lived in the same village as her, and described her as 'mad'. When I met her, she was unable to communicate; she spoke incoherently, and was unable to understand and follow my questions and conversations. I was told that she had received some healthcare but no clinical diagnosis for what her family believed to be a mental disorder. After interviews with Nomabali and her family, I consulted two psychiatrists, who, based on my description of her, concluded that she probably suffered from a severe mental disorder with psychotic features. This might, they suggested, be dementia, substance-induced psychotic disorder, schizophrenia, a mood disorder, or a psychosis due to a medical condition. Nomabali's story illustrates how it literally 'takes a village', not only to raise a child, but in this case to care for an elderly woman suffering from a severe mental disorder. As we describe in this case study, this involves a complex web of care and a multitude of interconnected care activities, care providers and care receivers within the family, household, village, community and region.[1]

In Madwaleni and similar African communities, where ubuntu philosophy is widely discussed and accepted, the obligation to care may extend far beyond immediate family members. As was discussed in Hochfeld, Chiba and Patel's case study 5.2, ubuntu emphasises collectivity rather than individualism, and the core of the philosophy is that humanness is expressed through social interaction. Individuals are often not seen as belonging to themselves or their families, but to society as a whole. While help-seeking and decision-making take on a largely individualistic approach in western biomedicine, in the context of ubuntu people may seek help and make decisions as a group (Cornell & Van Marle 2015).

Nomabali's household

Nomabali is a mother, grandmother, great-grandmother and great-great-grandmother. When she was younger, she worked at a luxury lodge near the village she lives in. Her family and neighbours described her as 'very clever' and able to speak English well. In her days working at the lodge, she earned a good income and was able to build a nice home with several houses and material possessions for herself and her family. Her husband had passed away some 20 years ago, and after his death she continued to work and care for the family. However, about five years prior to my visit to the family, two of Nomabali's three houses had burnt down in the middle of one night. No one knew what had happened, how the fire had started, or who or what had started it. No one was physically hurt, but Nomabali lost most of what she had worked so hard for. The police were informed but quickly closed the investigation; the cause of the fire was never resolved, and the family received no compensation. Two years after the fire, Nomabali's son passed away. He used to live with his family on the plot next to Nomabali. His widow, Sylvia, and other family members remained on that plot. Nomabali lived with her two great-granddaughters (20 and 16 years old), two great-grandsons (14 and 12 years old) and her great-great-granddaughter (8 months old). The oldest great-granddaughter, Vuyelwa (20 years old), was the head of the household, with primary responsibility of looking after her three younger siblings, her daughter, and her great-grandmother. Vuyelwa's mother was in Cape Town at the time of research looking for work; her grandmother was working at a hotel a few hours away; and her father and grandfather had both passed away. After the fire, Nomabali's immediate household of six people were left with only one functioning room of no more than 10 square metres. Inside this small room, they had a double bed, a single bed, a cabinet, and a table with cooking and eating utensils. In general, there is scarcity of sewage systems, running water and electricity in Madwaleni, especially in the area where Nomabali and her family live. The family had access to water only from rivers and streams; they had no electricity, and no formal sewage facilities. They prepared food on a paraffin cooker. They did not have any livestock, but they had a small garden where they grew vegetables.

The mental health of Nomabali

Vuyelwa explained that the mental health of her great-grandmother was bad. Two weeks before my first meeting with the family, Nomabali had had a seizure, and had been admitted to Madwaleni Hospital:

> Doctors don't see what's wrong. She doesn't have a pressure [high blood pressure], and she doesn't have a sugar diabetes. But she start fitting [having seizures], and it's not normal. What happened is that she was in good position before. Three years ago she was fine, five years ago was a burning of two houses that side, and since then her health start being not normal.

My granny [Nomabali] was not in the burning houses, but after that we noticed that it hurt her in the heart and in the mind ... The fire burnt all her goods. She was just staying [remaining] with the goods that were in that house we were in [when the fire happened – the house that did not burn down]. Those goods she tries them [earned them] with a lot of work. She was working, and when she stopped working at the hotel, saying that 'I have the goods now', it burnt. That's why she just become like this. It's the sadness of losing her things. And she is scared it will happen again.

Vuyelwa and Sylvia both explained that immediately after the fire, they noticed changes in Nomabali's behaviour. She spent most of her time for the first two years alone in her garden, avoiding other people, and she slept very little. Two years after the fire – around the time that Nomabali's son, Sylvia's husband, passed away – things changed further. Sylvia believed that the death had triggered Nomabali's deterioration: she didn't sleep at night; she wandered around aimlessly talking and singing to herself; and she was scared of people and her own reflection. When she saw herself in the mirror she became angry, as she thought the 'person' in the mirror had stolen her clothes and her things. She ceased to recognise her family and various friends, and become violent and aggressive when they tried to wash her, or when they lit the fire to cook. She also became confused, mixing strange ingredients when she was cooking, and urinating in the kitchen.

Caring for Nomabali

When I met Nomabali, she had required care and support from others for several years. Vuyelwa received some support from Sylvia and other family members outside the immediate household, but she was Nomabali's main caregiver. Vuyelwa's work included cooking; cleaning; working in the garden; looking after her younger siblings, her daughter and Nomabali; buying food and necessities; ensuring the health (seeking healthcare) for all members of the household; and more. Being head of the household and main caregiver took up all of her time. The immediate household survived primarily on Nomabali's old-age pension, CSGs, and some financial support from the extended household, particularly Vuyelwa's mother and grandmother.

Nomabali received support for all daily occupational activities, including personal care, and others undertook household chores and provided income to the household. With what were the best intentions, Nomabali's family had 'relieved' her of her chores and duties, believing that they were helping her. This may have been true. However, meaningful and adapted participation has been highlighted as key for an individual to flourish and prosper (Pereira & Whiteford 2013). Thus, the family's care may have been restricting her. As Eva Kittay et al. (2005) argue, good care is about providing care when it is needed, and refraining from providing care that interferes with people's freedom to exercise their capabilities and their own agency.

Seeking public healthcare

Two years after the fire, and three years before I met them, Nomabali's family had decided to seek assistance for her unusual behaviour. Health services in Madwaleni include a secondary hospital with 180 beds, which serves a population of more than 250 000, as well as seven primary healthcare clinics and one health centre spread evenly throughout the hospital catchment area. Owing to poor quality of the roads and frequent flooding, some clinics become unavailable to parts of the community for large parts of the year. The clinics are nurse run, with nursing assistants and community health workers in support. The clinics are severely understaffed and overworked. Lack of vehicles and ambulance services at the hospital, clinics and health centre limit the transportation of patients to and between health facilities. This also prevents staff from providing outreach services. When people experience mental-health problems and decide to seek healthcare for these, they first have to visit their local clinic. At the clinic they find staff with limited or no skills in recognising or diagnosing mental illness, and lack of appropriate medication. Most patients with mental illness come to the hospital in a very bad condition – escorted, tied up or held down, brought in by family members because of violent or aggressive behaviour, and viewed as a danger to themselves or to others. The most severe patients can be admitted to the general ward, where they can stay for a maximum of 72 hours for observation and treatment. In the general ward, medical conditions are mixed, and so psychiatric patients are admitted among other patients. They are most likely to be treated with sedatives or anti-psychotic medication. Relatives are often requested to stay with them, because of the layout of the ward, the many other patients, and the fact that hospital staff are unable to stay with the psychotic patient at all times.

Getting Nomabali to the hospital is costly and time consuming for the family. They have to rent a car with a driver for a day, which costs R400. Because Nomabali cannot go alone, someone has to accompany her. Getting there takes about one hour by car, at best; during rainy periods it takes longer, as the quickest road to the hospital floods and becomes impassable. At the hospital people are given appointment dates, which means that on that date they can be seen at any time, or not at all if the doctors do not have time to see all the patients before the hospital closes at 5.30 p.m. Patients will then be seen first thing the following morning, and will have to sleep overnight on the benches or the floors of the hospital. The local clinic is closer to Nomabali's home, but it is still quite costly to reach – again with a taxi, costing R18 per person one way. Over the years, Nomabali has been to the local clinic and to the hospital several times, usually accompanied by either Vuyelwa or Sylvia. Sylvia explained:

> There was nothing identified and recognised by the clinic. There was no pressure, hypertension, no sugar diabetes, there was no headache. They couldn't see anything. She was continuous doing things wrong, but when they testing her on those things and urinate [urine test] they couldn't see anything. But the only thing they failed to notice is that she must be a bit mad, but they don't know what should be the source of it. They did see that there could be problem in her mind, but they didn't see what could be the source of it. They advise us that we should repeat go to the clinic, and maybe it would be noticed what was the source. They gave her sleeping tablets and Panado; just for headaches. She didn't have headaches, but because she was a bit mad, you know mixing talking, so maybe they were just giving her such tablets.

Nomabali took the medication described by Sylvia every day for three years, but it seemed to make no difference in her behaviour. At the last visit to the hospital, Nomabali was prescribed some new pills: Haloperidol (an anti-psychotic) and thiamin (a vitamin-B supplement). They were not told what the medication was for, or if there were side effects, but just that Nomabali should take the pills. The first time I met the family was a few weeks after this last visit to the hospital. At that point, Vuyelwa felt that the pills had made no difference to her great-grandmother's behaviour. On my next visit, however, about a week later, the family felt that Nomabali was less aggressive and less confused. Towards the end of my three-week period knowing the family, Nomabali was visibly better. She spoke more coherently, and she seemed less scared and much less confused. She recognised people who she had not been able to recognise previously.

Vuyelwa wished that staff from the clinic or the hospital would pay visits to her great-grandmother, instead of making the family travel to the hospital every month. It was difficult and expensive for them to move Nomabali. She also wished that there had been a psychologist who could have visited Nomabali after the fire, someone 'that could take these things away from her heart. Then she couldn't be like this.'

The complex web of care

Most care starts at household level, where care decisions are made. Sometimes the care provided is poor, or less than optimal. However, as we see in Nomabali's household, overall choices about care are a matter of practical decision-making, based on the few choices available to them, with the overall aim of survival for the household. Optimal care becomes secondary, if that, to survival, and competing care demands within the immediate and extended household compromise the quality of care, and the livelihood and wellbeing of the family and the household as a unit. In Nomabali's case, various members of the immediate and extended household had different care responsibilities. Because Vuyelwa was the head of the household and responsible for the everyday care of Nomabali and the rest of the household, she dropped out of school. While Vuyelwa had the day-to-day responsibility of the household and of caring for Nomabali, her mother and grandmother – both working a few hours away – provided care by contributing to the income to the household. Nomabali's daughter-in-law, Vuyelwa's aunt, also helped care for Nomabali. Outside the immediate and extended household, the family received care from formal structures of care – the clinic and the hospital. They also received financial care from the government in terms of the various grants on which they depended for survival.

Health providers in Madwaleni had the impression that family- and community-support systems were good in the area, and that families genuinely wanted to help and care for sick family members as best as they could. Some attributed this to the ethics of ubuntu as a component of local culture. However, there may be both positive and negative aspects to ubuntu. While it is generally presented as a positive and inclusive philosophy in the literature, Dan Goodley and Leslie Swartz (2016) question this uncritical presentation. In the interdependent and collective nature of ubuntu, obligations and responsibilities follow in terms of who is obliged to carry out certain care activities, although this is not always the case (Manderson et al. 2016a). Vuyelwa has the obligation to be the main carer for the household in general as well as for her great-grandmother, and this has enormous negative implications for her own life and her dreams. Vuyelwa explained the impact of her great-grandmother's poor mental health:

> It has changed us because if she was not like this, I would not be responsible for this household. She would be responsible. Even my mother, she is supposed to stop working from now, because next year I will go to school, so no one will be responsible. So my mother will come back so I can go to school. My mother becomes depressed after the granny is like this. She is worried, and call every time, that 'how is mommy?' She wants to come back home.

Throughout this book, we have repeatedly referred to migration as impacting on families: first migration of men under apartheid, and now, with changing employment opportunities, migration of women who move from family settings to find work and generate an income to support others. We have paid little attention, however, to individual immigrants, communities of immigrants, the households which they establish or join, and how they provide and receive care (but see Mlotshwa and Merten's case study 2.5, Huschke's case study 3.4). Most migrants from within South Africa and beyond have limited choice in the kinds of work that they can find, the conditions of work and of living, the support systems that are available, or their access to formal healthcare. This limitation is especially marked for people who are working, or living without formal work, and who lack documents to prove citizenship or residency – preconditions for many services (see Blackie's case study 3.3). But an immigrant, whether from another part of South Africa or from another country, from the continent of Africa or beyond, is particularly vulnerable when alone and sick or frail.

In the following case study (6.4), based on the first author's extended ethnographic fieldwork, Linda Musariri and Eileen Moyer turn to the life and death circumstances of immigrant men. Migration, they suggest, disrupts gender norms, as men may have no option but to care for others when they are away from wider kin networks and when no women are available and able to undertake care work. The emotional and physical work of care in most settings is gendered, as was already considered in Chapter 4. Musariri and Moyer draw on the stories of two men who took on caregiving responsibilities, so going against such gender norms. These two men – Roby and Kudzai – were participants in an ethnographic study on masculinities in Johannesburg. While much of the research took place at Uncle Roby's Corner, located in the neighbourhood of Hillbrow, the authors also conducted in-depth interviews and had many informal conversations with men and women elsewhere in Johannesburg.

The two men are from different backgrounds and became caregivers in different circumstances: Roby (from Ghana), stepped up to provide an older Ghanaian man with care and support through to his death; Kudzai (from Zimbabwe), became the caregiver for his mother-in-law while her daughter, Kudzai's wife, continued to work. Both men had little choice but to provide personal care for people they considered family; pragmatics and affect combined to invert the conventions of gendered care.

Case study 6.4

Death and migrant communities of care

Linda Musariri and Eileen Moyer

Migration can shift gender dynamics, gender roles and traditional family structures. Here, we draw on the stories of two men who took on caregiving responsibilities, going against such gender norms. Both men found themselves in similar predicaments resulting from their being migrants living far from home, with limited kin networks to call upon in times of need.

His brother's keeper

Roby runs a makeshift stand at Uncle Roby's Corner, where he repairs shoes and sells ice cream to appreciative locals in a part of Johannesburg well known for its high levels of crime and violence. Located within the compound of a church, the corner was frequented by people looking to escape the hectic pace of the city. Passing through for a few minutes or hanging around for the whole day, over time some of the regulars developed bonds resembling kinship. This seemed to be especially so for migrants with limited family networks in South Africa. Despite its proximity to a church, not everybody who visited the corner was a churchgoer or even a customer of Roby's. Rather, most just seemed to enjoy hanging around: men, women, children, Muslims, Christians, traditionalists, police, professionals and unemployed, South Africans and foreigners from all over. A core group of regulars – all men – seemed to always be there, talking with one another and 'bird watching' (admiring women walking by). Despite the diverse backgrounds and nationalities of the men at Uncle Roby's Corner, they forged a sort of brotherhood, advising and caring for one another in ways that challenged their family and gender norms.

Roby, a 40-year-old Ghanaian man, was married to a South African woman and had been in South Africa for more than 10 years when we met him. He started repairing shoes when he was 28. Like most migrants, he had come to South Africa looking for better economic opportunities, but struggled to find a job. He resorted to fixing people's shoes in the streets, a trade of which he was at first ashamed. But, over the years, he expanded his shoe-repair business to include a phone shop and tuck shop where he sold his famous ice cream, sweets, snacks, toilet paper and airtime. He also had a machine for pay-as-you-go electricity. He often sold to people on credit – especially children with insufficient money for ice cream. It wasn't always clear how he made a profit. Although he sometimes complained about some people not paying, he was generally cheerful, laughing and talking even with those who owed him money.

Sometimes Roby would talk quietly with a friend, presumably offering counselling or some sort of advice. When asked about his seemingly natural ability to attract people, he replied: 'I am a prince from the Ashanti tribe, my father was a king. So, wherever I go, whether Libya or South Africa, I find people coming to me for help. It is my duty to take care of my people.' His royal heritage was reason enough for Roby to feel obligated to take care of the people around him – giving them freebies, or credit, or lending an empathetic ear. Despite being from Ghana, he would identify the people surrounding him as 'his' people – even the South Africans. Roby's acts of care extended beyond the corner, as first became apparent one windy morning in August 2017 when Linda arrived at the corner to find him absent.

She arrived at 10 a.m., but she found only Malume – a regular who occasionally helped Roby with the stall – there, standing alone by the gate next to the unopened stall. It was quite unusual to find only one man at the corner. Where was Roby? Had something horrible happened? Had he been shot dead, like another man who had lived in the neighbourhood and had recently been shot simply because he was a foreigner?

Malume said that Roby was late because he had to 'take care of some business', but offered no further elaboration. When Roby finally arrived, he looked distraught. He and Malume went about opening up the stall, and getting his stock, chairs and tables from the back room behind the church. Once the stall was open, Roby sat down and spoke about his morning. A Ghanaian friend whom Roby had been caring for over the previous weeks had finally succumbed to an illness. Roby had been giving updates on his progress every day for weeks, fondly referring to his friend as Baba, or father; coming from the same country, they had become good friends and had often shared a Ghanaian meal. Although they were quite close, Roby knew nothing about the man's family, other than that they were not available to take care of him when he fell critically ill. On the day he died, Baba had called Roby, asking him to bring him *fufu* and goat soup, a Ghanaian delicacy. Roby said Baba seemed strong and in a happy mood; he had thanked Roby for honouring his wish and taking care of him. Roby did not dwell on this gesture, but a few minutes after leaving his house that morning, Roby had received a call from a neighbour informing him that Baba had died.

Over the next couple of days Roby tried to contact Baba's family in Ghana, posting messages on Facebook and WhatsApp. Meanwhile, he stood in as an official relative to facilitate the paperwork required for Baba's burial, identified him at the mortuary, and went to the police station and the hospital to sign so that the body could be released. Just before the burial, he learned that Baba had a daughter living and working in South Africa. Neither the daughter nor Baba knew that the other was in Johannesburg, but she showed up just in time for the burial and took her father's belongings.

It was clear that it was not easy for Roby to look after and bury a 'father' who was also a stranger in many regards. He was caring for and mourning someone who was like kin to him. Despite struggling, Roby refused to talk to a counsellor, insisting he was fine. He described the care he gave to Baba, both preceding and following his death, as obligatory: 'Because we are in a foreign land with no mother, father, brother or sister, I became his brother. He had no one to look after him when he was sick, so I had to take care of him.' Being away from home redefined family ties for Roby and Baba, turning them into kin, responsible for one another.

How Roby cared for Baba highlights particular dynamics pertaining to kinship and family among migrants in South Africa. The fact that Baba lived in the same city as his daughter without either of them knowing was not very unusual. Neither was it unusual for Baba to forge new kinship bonds with Roby. Roby felt it was his responsibility to stand in as Baba's family at his death, but he would never have done so in Ghana. Migration, particularly among people who were economically marginal, has the potential to rupture family ties while facilitating the formation of new ties. Migration also shaped the gender of care relations. If Baba had been in Ghana, his daughter or another female relative would have been responsible for looking after him when he was sick. The task certainly would not have fallen to someone – a male – outside the family. Although it is true that Roby's values and sense of responsibility as a 'prince' crossed the borders with him, princes are rarely, if ever, asked to provide physical care for their male friends in Ghana, even those they call Baba.

When culture is irrelevant

In a situation similar to Roby's, Kudzai – a Zimbabwean professional in his mid-thirties living in Johannesburg – found himself undertaking care for his mother-in-law, something which would never have happened in Zimbabwe:

> It was not easy, because it's not just about the fact that she was my mum-in-law but because she was sick. That's the first hurdle; it's not easy to look after any sick person. Culture is irrelevant when you have no option. So I had to do it because, except for my wife in the later stages, nobody seemed to care. There is one moment that stays in my memory when my wife was away, and she, my mum-in-law, vomited, and I had to wipe her.

We did not interact with Kudzai on a daily basis as we did with Roby. But Kudzai was an excellent storyteller and, in interviews, he provided Linda with many details about his struggle to provide good care for his mother-in-law. Talking about picking up his mother-in-law from the airport, he recounted how he waited for more than two hours, wondering the whole time why it was taking her so long to come out. When she finally emerged, Kudzai was perplexed to see her in a wheelchair, escorted by an airport attendant. Finally, he understood why she had taken so long. The last time he had seen her, she had been able to walk on her own; he had not known that she had gotten so sick. He knew that over the past few months her health had deteriorated immensely, to the point where he and his wife, Sheila, had decided to bring her to South Africa to access better treatment. In addition to diabetes mellitus, she had recently been diagnosed with kidney failure. His wife was the only female child in her family and, although she has three married brothers, she was expected to care for her mother. Kudzai and Sheila first hired a domestic helper to look after their mother in Harare, but as the illness intensified they decided to bring her to Johannesburg to monitor her more closely.

Kudzai told how he took his mother-in-law's small black suitcase from the polite airport attendant, while also taking over the wheelchair. He recalled how unsettled he was pushing her towards the parking lot, and how he absentmindedly asked how the trip was and how things were back home. Kudzai said that despite being completely up to date on the news from Zimbabwe, he felt compelled to make conversation. He noted how frail his mother-in-law sounded when responding, telling him that things were not changing for the better, that there were still cash-flow shortages, that commodities in the shops had become very expensive, and that corruption was commonplace. She told him that the political landscape was quite shaky, and that political violence was rampant though not spoken of. These were things he already knew. Kudzai said that despite her being homebound due to her illness, she spoke with confidence, as though she had first-hand experience. Maybe this was why he had not discerned the severity of her condition from their phone calls.

Kudzai recounted that he could hardly hear her responses as various thoughts were racing through his mind. Given the state of her health, who was going to look after her, particularly since his wife was out of town on a business trip and would be away for a while? His heart quivered at the thought of having to provide care to her. Worse still, what would people say when they saw him carrying her around, feeding her, and so on? Back in Zimbabwe, a son-in-law is not even supposed to sit near his mother-in-law, let alone touch her. Yet he saw no choice. 'Culture is irrelevant when you have no option,' he said. He noted that being in Johannesburg, away from home, away from nosy relatives and neighbours, made it a bit easier; in Johannesburg, no one really cared if he broke the taboo of touching his mother-in-law.

A few days later his wife returned, but Kudzai decided to continue to help to care for his mother-in-law, saying he could not let his wife 'do it on her own'. For six months Kudzai and Sheila took turns caring for her. Both had demanding jobs, so they had to make a schedule, including visiting her in the hospital when she was admitted. Kudzai found himself doing unusual chores for a man in his position – feeding her, cleaning her, helping her get out of bed, or helping her to walk around the ward. Public hospitals in South Africa expect relatives, usually female, to attend to daily care needs while hospital staff focus on medication. For Kudzai's mother-in-law, who spoke Shona, this was difficult. While isiNdebele, the other main language spoken in Zimbabwe, is similar to isiZulu, Shona is not easily understood by most South Africans, and Shona speakers cannot understand isiZulu. Kudzai, like many Zimbabweans, spoke both Shona and isiNdebele, and so could converse with the nurses at the hospital and translate for his mother-in-law. His presence was therefore indispensable.

At first Kudzai was quite uncomfortable. He could feel other people in the hospital – patients, nurses and visitors – staring, but there was nothing he could do. Sheila could not quit her job to focus on her mother. They had bills for which they were jointly responsible, more so with his mother-in-law in hospital. They had to pay school fees, rent and food, and regularly send money home to his parents and other relatives. They had to work as a team. If he was not at work or at the hospital, he was at home looking after their four children; the same was true for

Sheila. The only time Kudzai took a break was when Sheila's sisters-in-law briefly visited. He explained:

> I did all this because I love my wife; I just wanted to support her. While it was odd at first, I had to learn to be strong. You end up doing things that you normally do not do. However, I felt it was an honour to do that for my mother-in-law who to me is like my mother. I know my culture says other things, but I didn't mind doing it as a man. Of course in the hospital I could only see women doing the work that I was doing, but I didn't mind doing it since my wife was at work.

Kudzai referred to his mother-in-law as being 'like his own mother', which is quite uncommon in Shona culture, which has distinct names for the two relations: *amai* for mother and *ambuya* for mother-in-law. Being in a foreign land, however, Kudzai improvised to adapt to the situation. He decided to care for his mother-in-law, doing things he would not have done at home to support his wife, given that they did not have a wider kin network to draw support from.

Kudzai's story is similar to Roby's in that both men cared for people they considered to be kin when no other options were available. Although both men took on the responsibility of providing physical care, despite contrary gendered cultural norms, we hesitate to argue that their behaviour be read as evidence of changing gender norms or evidence of questioning of the status quo. Rather, a combination of imposition and chance led each of them to become a caregiver for older people. They both found themselves in situations without better options. With no woman – daughter, sister or mother – free to take care of the sick elderly person, they did it.

In a foreign land with minimal or no kin support, some African male migrants find themselves in caregiving roles, looking after children or doing household chores while women are at work. Some might label men like Roby and Kudzai as responsible men – men who should be seen role models. Neither Kudzai nor Roby celebrated this behaviour as enlightened, feminist, or even normal, and men's taking up care work does not necessarily translate to gender equality. Migration may disrupt gender norms, but, also, a man may simply have no option but to care when he is away from wider kin networks and no women are able to do the work.

Popular sentiment and state discourse emphasise the role of the family in meeting the healthcare needs of those who are young and dependent, have limits to their capability, are ill, or are elderly and frail. But sometimes households and families break down. In small households especially, a single event can unsettle the balance of care. One member may need to leave others alone to find work, perhaps without recognising the consequences of doing this. Householders who have undertaken most care – sometimes economic, physical and emotional – may become ill themselves and be unable to continue care work. The loss of adult household members through migration or death – including as a consequence of HIV but also due to sudden events such as accidents, suicide, homicide or a stroke – leave indelible dents in household resilience. Many causes can undo the stability of the household and the predictability of family-based care when previously it had been in place; for example, economic constraints and deprivation, loss of work, sudden hospitalisation, social upheaval, violence or growing isolation for any reason. Variations in external social-support systems – including those of unrelated friends, neighbours and non-resident kin – impact on the health and wellbeing of all householders. Good care, in these contexts, is shaped by chronic illness, poverty and scarce resources.

While community health workers and healthcare providers at primary health-care centres may be aware of difficulties in some households, time and resources constrain their capacity to respond in a sustained manner. Often, the increased hardships individuals experience from catastrophic changes in circumstances, or as a result of the slow grinding down of resources, go unnoticed. In the following case study (6.5), Jessica Ruthven focuses on a newly formed residential-care unit that also provides home-based care to people on a waiting list for admission. Her ethnographic field research, a combination of extended observation and interviews conducted in 2016 and 2017, focused on one such centre based in a small rural village in northeast Mpumalanga Province. The centre was was founded in 2013 by a local man, Akani, aged 21 at the time, whose concern about older family members and others without access to personal care led him to open it. The small unit he started was intended as an institution providing respite and ongoing care, with people taken there if their health problems exceeded the ability of family members to provide adequate care at home. The decision for them to move into the centre was often made through consensus with family members. Two years after Akani founded it, the centre had moved to other buildings and grown from 12 beds to 100. While its aim was to provide quality care for people without home support, it also became a resort for crisis care. In this case study, Ruthven questions the role of non-state actors in providing care for people who are frail and/or aged, while she raises the possibility that people may need to make conscious decisions about the care and support of others outside their own families.

Case study 6.5

'Suffering grannies'

Jessica Ruthven

When you think of a household, what image comes to mind? If you were like the upper-class, female, white South African neighbour I asked, you might answer as she did: 'My children and my home.' What associations do you make when you see the word 'family'? If you were from the USA, middle class, and watched a lot of television as a kid, you might think of a small, brick house with a man, a woman, two children, and a dog playing in a grassy yard. What do you feel when you think about the notion of 'healthcare'? If you were like my friend Buhle, a 36-year-old African woman living in Orlando East, Soweto, whose mother was recently hospitalised, you might respond as she did: 'Stress.'

Between July 2016 and March 2017, I spent three months in a small, rural village in South Africa exploring how people in the community defined these terms and enacted them in everyday life, and how these definitions and practices compared to those of the staff and clients in the village's newly formed residential-care centre. After speaking with a range of people across gender and age categories, it became apparent that village residents' answers to my questions diverged in important ways from the kinds of relationality I saw at the care home. To address this and the impacts of changing family composition and household structure, I examine what people think and feel about getting older and how those ideas are shaped by context. I focus on providing an account of the ways in which people think about ageing in rural South Africa, and how they conceptualise 'good care' in contexts of chronic illness, poverty and scarce resources.

Village pressures and suffering grannies

Central to gaining a picture of how people in the village defined households or good healthcare is an understanding of how they experience life in the village, including its hardships. When we chatted, people expressed opinions about pressures, and noted that life was unpleasant – as it had always been. Every person with whom I spoke argued that few changes had been made since democratisation in 1994. 'We were struggling before 1994,' Xaniseka, a 64-year-old woman born in the village, stated. 'And we are *still* struggling.'

The only major changes in the last two decades anyone could identify were the very new addition of the residential-care home and a high school completed the previous year. None of the houses had running water, and all used an unreliable community pump for water. Sometimes, people were left without drinking water unless they could afford to buy it from the nearest grocery store, a 40-minute drive away by minibus taxi. Transportation was also a problem. No roads in or leading to the village were tarred. Even the main road became a dangerous and muddy mess of potholes after rain, often responsible for 'breaking people's cars', although few people could afford to own vehicles, and those who did could not always use them. Owing to the remoteness of the village, the minibus taxis servicing it ran irregularly, impeding people's ability to travel anywhere quickly.

Residents spoke of water and transport in conjunction with discussions of access to healthcare, food and education. The village lacked a health clinic, but instead had a 'visiting site' with space for bi-monthly mobile health-clinic visits. It also lacked shops. Other factors cited as contributing to hardship included high rates of unemployment, heat, drought and high rates of death from HIV and AIDS. In conjunction with structural problems, the residents identified health issues of major concern: obesity, hypertension, stroke, arthritis, diabetes, dementia and stress. Combining these concerns, Nhlamulo, an 86-year-old HIV-positive woman, said:

> We have no shops. If you want to get groceries, even something little like soap, sometimes you wait over an hour for a taxi to go to the town with shops – and you already had to walk far to get to that station. Maybe you're sick, tired, have grandchildren at home to take care of, and it's hot, and maybe the roads are mud. And then you have only some little money, from the old-age pension, to get your mealie meal, sugar, washing powder. It's just not enough.

When I asked about hardships related to older people particularly, people expressed concern about what they called 'elder abuse', or more colloquially, 'suffering grannies'. In describing this, they talked about people being emotionally abused, degraded, subjected to sexual violence, or addressed in abusive language. They told stories about people who had their social-grant money repeatedly stolen by family members or strangers; people who were left alone for weeks at a time to starve; and those who were isolated and lonely. This narrative held strong resonance in the community, despite the fact that few people were able to provide more than one example of a person they knew who fitted this 'suffering granny' profile.

Community understandings: 'household' and 'good care'

In this context, how people conceive of both 'households' and taking 'good care' of ageing populations is important. By and large, people defined a household in terms of a dwelling that housed a family. In turn, a family was most often defined as a person's children, siblings, parents and sibling's (often brother's) children. When they spoke of caring for ageing populations, people overwhelmingly indexed 'good care' of the elderly as feeding them, bathing them, taking them to the toilet when requested, not shouting at them, taking them to the clinic, and taking them to the residential-care centre if necessary. Since the care centre had been established only a year earlier, this latter example was a recent addition.

For instance, according to Mulweri, a 76-year-old man who was born locally, 'good care' occurred when a family member hired someone to cook, wash clothes, clean the house, or do any tasks an elderly person required. George, a 58-year-old HIV-positive man who was born in Mozambique but had moved to the village in 1978, echoed Mulweri's views. However, George framed them in more reciprocal and familial terms: 'If a man has a wife, she will take good care of him by bringing him cold drinks, cooking for him, bathing him, cleaning the house, anything. And he will do the same for her if she is sick or too old.'

Most women with whom I spoke, aged from 54 to 86, concurred; they defined 'good care' as cooking, bathing and cleaning for a person, washing their clothes, feeding them, taking them to the clinic when necessary, and giving them correct medication. Tengisa, a 65-year-old woman who had moved to the village in 1964, mentioned many of these tasks but added what she considered necessary qualities: patience and dedication. Nonisa, a 59-year-old resident, noted: 'There are a lot of grannies here, but they have people to take care of them, and they're mostly doing okay. The ones who weren't okay, they went to the old-age home.'

Residential-care home

After two years of fund-raising and research, including trips to the facilities of four 'old-age homes' in Gauteng Province, Akani started a volunteer-led residential-care home operating out of a house donated by a local woman who had moved to a neighbouring province and abandoned her village home. Akani recruited volunteers from his church congregation to act as staff, and their care home opened in 2013. As the number of residents slowly increased, Akani decided they needed to expand, and in October 2014 he resumed active fundraising.

Eventually, Akani secured land and sufficient funds to build a new residential-care home and hire additional staff to help care for the increased population of residents. They moved into the new place in August 2016. The new facility included a fenced property with a security stand, a main building near the entrance, a smaller building at the back, and a bore hole which provided running water. The main building housed the majority of residents in three large rooms, two with bathrooms with flush toilets and fully tiled shower areas. The main building had a covered veranda, a room for sick residents, separate offices for a nurse and manager, a dining room and a kitchen. The smaller building contained laundry facilities and two rooms to house additional male residents.

At the time of my fieldwork, the residential-care home accommodated around 45 registered residents from villages across the province. It also housed 17 temporary residents with dementia-related issues, who were found wandering alone elsewhere in the province and had family in the study area; they were taken by various village police to the centre for care. Services for residents included basic nursing care, palliative care, frail care and hospice care. While four registered residents were HIV-positive and one had epilepsy, the centre catered mainly to people with dementia, stroke, diabetes, hypertension and disability.

Despite its expansion, the care home was understaffed and underfunded. Akani, 25 years old in 2017, remained the manager and employed a project manager for administrative tasks, a senior nurse, three kitchen staff, two cleaners, three security guards, and a rotating roster of about 10 caregivers. While I was there, a second nurse was hired. Although the centre's policy was to have eight caregivers working each day shift, usually only three or four caregivers were on duty at any time. Still, people worked there in the absence of other employment opportunities and out of a genuine concern for the elderly. Among current staff, some had certificates in ancillary healthcare from a local college, others had limited training from the Department of Health, and at least three caregivers had no training.

Care centre understandings: 'household' and 'good care'

Contrary to the opinions of some community members, the centre was not primarily an institution where people went if they had no family. Rather, people were taken if their health issues exceeded the ability of family members to provide adequate care at home. With some exceptions, residents noted that they had decided to move into the centre through consensus with family members. When asked, residents largely defined a 'household' in the same terms as community members and initially expressed similar ideas about what constituted 'good care' for ageing populations. However, after probing, some expanded on their notions of care in what they called the 'old-age home' context.

Most residents expressed satisfaction with the kind of care they received at the residential-care home. For example, Drondro, a 70-year-old man with dementia who had been at the residential-care home for a year, and Dzunani, a 60-year-old man who had arrived three months earlier, noted that good care meant giving residents plenty of food, water, and clothes; making sure they got to the toilet safely; and ensuring they were able to sleep well at night. Sana, a 56-year-old woman who came to the centre in November 2016 after a stroke, noted: 'They treat me well here, and it feels like home. They cook for me, bathe me, and give me as much food as I want. To take good care of someone is to treat them as your own mother. These caregivers are young, but they are good.' Another resident, Nyakwavi, held a different opinion. Partially blind, she had been at the residential-care home for three years, first in the old premises and then in the new facility:

> The old place had better caretakers, but this new place is nicer and has showers and flush toilets. But the new caretakers aren't gentle when they take me to the shower. They don't care about me. They'd even leave me here if I fell down! To me, bathing and cooking for someone equals good care. The kitchen staff, now, *they* take care of me.

According to staff members, 'good care' for the residents clustered around the few key actions cited also by community members: bathing, feeding, giving residents correct medication, helping them to bed or to the toilet, and helping them maintain hygiene. Several staff members cited providing proper diet, nutrition, physical exercise, and a clean environment as important elements of care. Although people first mentioned physical concerns, the residents and staff at the residential-care home often underscored other aspects of caregiving, such as patience with residents, speaking to them with kindness and respect, chatting with them to stave off boredom, providing company by listening to their stories and laughing at their jokes, noticing when residents seemed unwell, and, as one staff member said, generally making sure 'their minds are not upset'.

Residential-care homes: A different kind of 'household'

Poverty and poor infrastructure remain a burden in the village and throughout the district. They shape health and wellbeing and contribute to the ways in which people understand what it means to take good care of another person. National social-welfare grants are an integral source of income in this region, and people aged 60 and over have become important to household economies through contributions made by their pensions (Schatz & Madhavan 2011). While this might motivate some families to resist sending an elderly relative to a care centre, this was not so among the people with whom I worked. Instead, there was deep concern about the wellbeing of the elderly, and people of all ages often invoked an elderly person's health and comfort as paramount to considering their role in a household. This was articulated not just by people from the village, but also by the residents and staff members of the residential-care home from other villages across the province.

Although people in the community and residential-care home gave similar answers when asked what 'households' and 'good care' meant, there were crucial differences between households in the community and the types of relationality within the residential-care home. The reality of life at the residential-care home mirrored people's articulated understandings in some ways but differed markedly in others. For example, most people in the area live in multigenerational, extended family units on plots of land in close proximity (Madhavan & Brooks 2016), and households consist of a range of people related biologically or through kinship configurations.

For the community members with whom I spoke, taking 'good care' of ageing populations primarily signalled attending to their physical wellbeing, although older community members also cited spending time with grandchildren as important. In contrast, life at the residential-care home was characterised by the daily interaction of a large number of people – staff and residents – from disparate villages and across age cohorts. There was constant movement of people in and out of the care home as some residents recovered from illnesses and returned to their homes, others died, some left on short trips to visit family, and new residents moved into the facility. Residents had plenty of food, running water, and company to combat loneliness and boredom. The care relationships produced or enabled within this care-home environment were crucially built around friendship and companionship. Not all residents got along, and people bickered on a daily basis. However, this kept things interesting, and residents would pull me aside to share care-centre gossip.

The residential-care home is located in one of the most undeveloped villages in the Agincourt study site (mentioned in the introductory text preceding case study 6.2), and it contained a newly built residential-care centre. Originally intended to house the elderly of this village, it quickly became a home to people from across the sub-district, as there are no other such full-time residential-care centres. While it is not usually so depicted, the residential-care centre comprises a type of contemporary, dynamic South African household with a constantly shifting composition. Understanding it this way allows us to ask about new forms of care and care relations instantiated within this space, and how this type of institution meets evolving community needs in a rural context. It also provides a starting point for challenging our common-sense ideas about what comprises households and how we can think about them elsewhere in the world.

Death asks that families continue to perform as kin, and to make kinship with those who have died. In the immediacy of a death, whether sudden or anticipated, regardless of the age of the person who has died, families converge. The urgency of the present at times overrides other family agendas; at times it exposes the clefts that separate individual members or groups of kin. In hospital settings, increasingly family members are asked to enact care by deciding when death might occur – through ceasing active treatment, for example. The manner of death, the care of the body, the burial and funeral are all moments to celebrate connected lives and expose their disconnections. Each ceremony and anniversary is an occasion, celebrated or not, for individuals to reflect and find comfort. Cemeteries provide a spatial focus for the effects of death on those who survive. Historically, these were largely segregated in South Africa, allowing (or enforcing) a sense of community identity shaped by social, economic and political circumstance.

Lorena Núñez Carrasco, in the case study that follows (6.6), turns our attention to the role of the cemetery among one group of South Africans – Chinese descendants – in honouring their own ancestors, in grieving for their most recently departed family members, and in remembering the history of families and the larger community of which they are a part. As she describes this, Chinese South Africans visit deceased family members buried at Newclare Cemetery, a previously segregated burial space in Johannesburg, twice a year. In her account, members of the Fu family visit the cemetery to clean the tombs, place flowers, and tell stories of those who they visit. Through these actions, members of the younger generation learn about the lives of their deceased relatives, their relations to the living, and the way they encountered death, and so develop a sense of family history. The cemetery visits and the caring for the deceased are animated by the perception of the wellbeing of the dead as deeply connected to that of the living. Núñez Carrasco describes caring for the dead as a form of caring for the living, with this burial space a site that evokes, for the living, a sense of place and belonging in post-apartheid South Africa. In unfolding these effects through the lens of care and the work of place and memory, she explores the ritualistic importance of connecting with the ancestors as animating the Chinese traditions in South Africa.

Case study 6.6

Caring for the dead

Lorena Núñez Carrasco

The size of the Chinese population in contemporary South Africa is unknown, but it numbers probably between 100 000 and 300 000 (Mung 2008). This is the result of migration in a first wave in the 1870s, then indentured miners who arrived from 1904 and were expatriated soon after, and a third wave of migration, primarily from Taiwan, in the 1980s. While the public display of Chinese cultural heritage – such as the celebration of the Chinese New Year and the culinary traditions offered by Chinese restaurants – are well known and part of South Africa's diverse cultural landscape, rituals related to ancestor veneration and the care of the dead are less well known.

Visiting cemeteries to commemorate the dead is common in South Africa, as in mainland China and elsewhere. Twice a year, Chinese celebrate *Qingming*, when families visit all the cemeteries in the city where members with the same clan name are buried. Family names were taken from the place from where the first generation of immigrants came, and are shared by all from the same locality in China; in the past, the clan name was important in the construction of solidarity in the Chinese South African community. Visitors burn incense and lay fresh flowers on the tombs. These occasions are normally followed by a shared meal in a restaurant. In addition to *Qingming*, individual families visit specific cemeteries at particular times in the year to commemorate the deaths of relatives – primarily patrilineal – and may also visit graves at other times for personal reasons, such as in preparation for a trip, before getting married, or at other important transitions in their lives.

I look at visits to Newclare Cemetery in Johannesburg by three generations of the Fu family, the family of my friend Jacquie, a second-generation Chinese South African. Between 2015 and 2017, I visited the cemetery on three occasions and participated in family gatherings; I conducted interviews with family members on cemetery visits, on ancestor veneration, and on their identity as Chinese South Africans.

In this case study, I ask the questions 'How do death rituals contribute to the construction of a Chinese South African identity?' and 'What is the relationship between caring for the living and caring for the dead?'

Newclare Cemetery

The Group Areas Act (No. 41 of 1950) and the Reservation of Separate Amenities Act (No. 49 of 1953), issued during the apartheid era, ruled on the use of land and control of space, regulating the bodies of both the living and the dead. Consequently, cemeteries were racially managed (Moyo et al. 2016), and until the 1950s, people were interred in separate cemeteries or in shared cemeteries divided into racially defined blocks. Newclare cemetery was founded in 1934 for all populations, and when the African section of the cemetery filled up, African people's burials were moved to other parts of the city. However, the cemetery reached full capacity only in the 1980s, by which time it was particularly known for its Chinese and Muslim sections, and as the final resting place of struggle heroes such as Walter Sisulu. Originating under apartheid, such old cemeteries are an ethnic enclave inhabited by the dead, whose presence becomes alive only in the stories that are told by the living who visit them. In these visits, second-generation Chinese South Africans pass on stories to those who are even younger, while they position themselves in relation to time and space, with respect to their past under apartheid and in relation to mainland China.

The Fu family

The Fu family visit the cemetery of Newclare in January each year to commemorate the death of the family patriarch, the grandfather who came from China to South Africa. They also visit Newclare in June to commemorate the death of Jacquie's brother, who died at a young age of a heart attack in the 1980s. But these are only two of those whose graves are visited on these occasions.

On 24 January 2015, I took part in the commemoration of the death of Jacquie's grandfather, who had died in 1972. There were nine of us, across three generations. Jacquie's father, in his eighties, was there. He had been born in China, and had migrated to South Africa at the age of 18 in 1948 to be reunited with his family. His daughters Sylvie and Bet, in their fifties, their spouses and partners, and two of the grandchildren in their twenties were also present. They were joined by Jacquie's cousin, whose wife was buried in this cemetery in the 1970s, and the cousin's sisters, who were visiting from Canada. Jacquie was not present, so I was guided by Sylvie, her sister, who introduced me to the family.

While gatherings among extended members of the clan name are not common, the Fu family still conveys a sense of being part of a same community of origin in their cemetery visits. The visit included the graves of the deceased family members in a patrilineal order, with two males from Jacquie's father's side as the central figures, but also including Jacquie's mother and the families her sisters have married into. We visited 16 graves in total. Starting with the grave of the patriarch, we continued in geographic order, visiting the deceased brother, then Jacquie's maternal grandparents, her mother's stepsister and so on. At each grave, flowers left from a previous visit were thrown away, new flowers and clean water were placed in clean vases, and the weeds were removed. As the fresh flowers were laid, each family member took turns to stand in front of the grave, and with their hands together at the centre of their chest, to bow three times.

As we walked around, tomb by tomb, each deceased person would be remembered and some details provided about their lives or the manner in which they died. The kinship relationship of the deceased with the living would be traced, so that the younger generation would know what relation existed between them. New biographical details triggered interest and surprise, sometimes incredulity, leading to efforts to confirm with each other veracity, until the new information could be corroborated. The tombs look alike – black marble tombstones with Chinese characters inscribed. Some graves were also adorned with Christian crosses or icons of saints. Others had no visible religious symbols. Sylvie's grandfather was a Buddhist, as is the case, she explained, for most of the older generation. Younger-generation Chinese, like Jacquie and Sylvie, became Catholic and attended Catholic schools.

The visits to the cemetery, I was told, are occasions to remember the lives and deaths of deceased relatives and members of clans. They are also occasions to remember a whole generation of Chinese people who lived through apartheid. Brief snapshots of their lives are specifically directed to the younger generation. As the stories are told, people add information if they knew a particular person, or give details that highlight what it meant for them to live in a racially segregated society. Jacquie would remember, for example, how her own father, a shopkeeper, had his shop right in front of the Pass Office in downtown Johannesburg, 'where all black people had to go to obtain permits.' She reflects on how curious this place was, as 'almost every black person in the city had to queue there to obtain a permit and would come to my dad's shop to have a meal.' She points out that the significance of these memories did not emerge until later in her life, when she became more politically aware and realised that her father's shop was placed at 'the heart of the apartheid'. Jacquie stresses how her parents' generation was not politicised: 'They simply would not talk about what their experiences were during the apartheid.' This first Chinese generation in South Africa endured the brunt of oppression and segregationist systems. As Yoon Jung Park has noted, 'Chinese became with very few exceptions, model citizens: law abiding, quiet, non-violent, non-confrontational, polite, educated and above all respectable' (2009: 58).

Jacquie reflects on her parents' stance, 'more concerned with survival and for their children to get a good education'. Today her parents still do not communicate much about the past; they are reluctant to engage in what it meant to live under apartheid. Moreover, second-generation Chinese still mostly speak Cantonese and are not fluent in English. Among the Fu family at the cemetery, Jacquie and her sisters Bet and Sylvie led these conversations.

Who will care for the dead in the future?

This is a question I posed to several members of the Fu family. At the time of our interview, Sylvie had been to the cemetery three times in a month, twice accompanying her partner Frederick's family and once with her own family. Sylvie feels the need to continue this tradition, to continue to embrace her parents' culture. She thinks that younger people do not understand the full meaning of these practices, nor do they have the knowledge, but they still have their parents around. Whether these practices will continue among the third generation remains in question.

Sylvie gives the example of her brother, who in Chinese patrilineal order should be the bearer of the tradition. But, she reflects, 'He never really encouraged his children much to participate, but the two sons now are grown-up … one nephew was in a relationship with someone who was a Jehovah['s] Witness who opposed to the visits to the cemeteries and so for a while he didn't come and never participated.' This nephew married a member of a well-known Chinese family who follows the traditions strictly, and he now joins the cemetery visits. Sylvie concludes, 'Being married to someone from a family that respects the Chinese tradition, it is quite likely that he and his brother will continue observing these traditions.' In Jacquie's view Sylvie has 'lately become much more Chinese than before', because of her relationship with Frederick, a Cantonese speaker also from a traditional family. Sylvie admires this, as her own mastery of the language is not strong even though her parents always spoke in Cantonese.

Despite patrilineal conventions, the women of the families sustain the tradition. Jacquie concludes that patriarchal structures may alter with women taking the lead: 'In an immigrant's situation it is about a traditional bearer rather than men or woman, and Bet is the traditional bearer in our family … she may say she doesn't know what is going to happen but she would do … she will do it.' The Fu sisters are the bearers of the tradition both in their own families and in the families into which they marry. Sylvie and Bet explain that when they married (men in the Chinese community), they fully participated in the cultural traditions of the families of their spouses, so that there would be times they wouldn't see their parents for months. Now, with grown-up children, they have come back to their own parents to join them in their death rituals. Bet says,

> It is now the girls' side of our family [accompanying the parents to their visits to the cemetery] and we do it because Mom and Dad … they are the first generation so we follow what they do. Every year they call us and we do it … whether we will continue the tradition? I can't say.

Sylvie adds, 'Well, for me … I am not sure what Bet will do, [but] because I am with Frederick now, and knowing his family and how he brought up his own child, I think I will continue with the tradition that is how I would like it … otherwise the custom will die.'

The question about authenticity is recurrent. Sylvie initially warned me, 'We are not the right family [to study Chinese traditions], we don't do it very well – other people stick to the tradition much more than us.' She now feels assured that Frederick's family will provide a source of certainty. Frederick joined us to discuss the differences in cemetery visits in China, and a younger woman was called in to tell us how is it done there, as she had recently been in China with her own parents. Frederick suggested we Google this for more information.

I asked the three sisters who they thought would carry on the tradition. Bet indicated that she can already anticipate the tradition fading: 'I will not force anybody; my children will definitely not carry on. They are so westernised they do not feel the relevance of this, it will definitely be lost on my side of the family, and that is sad … they are so caught up in their own lives.' Sylvie was more confident: 'If my daughter was here, she would jointly carry on with Bet's daughter.' As Bet's daughter, Mary, was around, I asked her directly. Mary laughed and responded: 'Well, we will do it for special occasions only because that is the way you do it.' Jacquie pushed her: 'When we die something will spark and they would feel the responsibility … but Mary, it's nothing more than what we do now … you would do it?' Mary replied: 'Not on my own …'

The cemetery provides the stage for three generations of Chinese South Africans to position themselves with regard to their identity. Park (2009) labelled the first of these generations as 'the older shopkeepers'; their South African-born children as 'fence-sitters' who benefitted from opportunities for upward mobility and social mixing; and the third generation as 'bananas' ('yellow outside, white inside') with little Chinese culture and who see themselves mainly as South Africans.

The Fu family presents a more nuanced picture in which the boundaries of cultural commitment are crossed in their cemetery visits. Chinese South Africans may move away from certain Chinese cultural traditions, but they may also return to embrace them as they accompany others or take the lead. As has been noted, members of these families are the bearers of this tradition, unconventionally taking the lead in what is generally characterised as a traditional patriarchal culture.

For Jacquie, Sylvie and Bet, these visits, and the spontaneous storytelling that took place around the headstones, served to mediate between the experiences of three generations: their own experiences as children of Chinese parents growing up under apartheid; the experiences of their children as 'born free' Chinese descendants in the new South Africa; and their grandparents' experiences as new immigrants. The cemetery visits are not only an encounter with the particular lives and biographies of deceased Fu family members, but are also encounters between generations who lived under apartheid. By caring for their graves of deceased family members, Jacquie, Sylvie and Bet continue to care for their elders, with the hope that others in turn will visit and lay flowers on their headstones.

Our aim in this chapter has been to examine sources of vulnerability and resilience within households when there is an increasing demand for care, especially with elderly householders, and to describe shifts in practice and care in the absence of strong family resources, as a result of migration, for instance, or changing family circumstance. Economic, personal, social and intellectual resources are spread unevenly within households, among families and across populations. They are also shaped by local resources within communities and districts. Access to support, and the availability of support, in providing care in a middle-class household is quite different to that available to a household in a remote village; the different circumstances of these households result in differences in the available options or limits, the affordability and capacity to pay, and knowledge about services that are available.

People share caregiving and supportive roles within and beyond households, and within and beyond conventional families and kinship ties. Demographic as well as economic changes in contemporary South Africa have forced, to some extent, a reworking of households and families. Family structures may deviate from community norms, and may be multigenerational households. Increasingly, with ageing, households include at least one member with extended care needs; as we have seen, the impact of caregiving can be mitigated within the household, kinship networks, social entrepreneurship (as in the case of the residential centre), and the wider community.

Note

1   Information about Nomabali, her life, mental disorder and care was obtained through in-depth interviews (with several family members, healthcare professionals and neighbours) and observations (in her home, in the community and at the hospital) conducted by Stine Hellum Braathen in 2012.

7 Families, care and support

Nolwazi Mkhwanazi and Lenore Manderson

Through kinship and residence, families and households connect and give meaning to lives. The rhythms and routines of daily life play out through these connections and in these settings. Families and households take care of basic human needs: food and shelter, reproduction, and social and daily production. This occurs whether the family is biologically based or chosen, heterosexual or otherwise, large or small, matrilineal or patrilineal, nuclear or extended. Likewise, households might draw their core members from marriage and blood ties, or they might be intentional, the members drawn together through love and affective ties. Households can be very small and stable, or extremely large and fluid, spreading and shrinking as personal circumstances, and domestic and local economics allow. Families provide practical and emotional ties for people to feel supported; households provide the settings in which these ties are lived out day by day. Beyond and within households, families provide the structures and resources for everyday life, and the context through which people manage intermittent, often minor but sometimes catastrophic, health, economic and other crises (Makiwane et al. 2017). They are at the heart of birth and death, health and illness. Within them, biology and sociality are intertwined, often inseparably.

In South Africa, we speak of ubuntu. Nelson Mandela and Desmond Tutu used ubuntu theologically, but the term has been popularised as foundational of humanity (Membe-Matale 2015). It is commonly used as a political philosophy, implicitly underpinning the Constitution and its values of social inclusion. But one of its translations into English – *I am because we are* – captures also the individual in relation to a family and a household, and conversely illustrates how the two are co-produced and conditional. Families and households exist only because of the individuals who constitute them, but equally, we exist because of families and households. Humans are deeply social beings, and must be so to come into being, survive and thrive. The institutions and networks of people that make up families and households, overlapping yet different, are central also to community and state-making. This is why governments and community-based organisations try to support them in different ways, through grants and local programmes, for instance, as some case-study authors have illustrated (see for example Patel et al. 2017a; Schatz et al. 2012; Schneider et al. 2008; Shenderovich et al. 2018).

Through the case studies woven through this book, we have examined people's desires and commitments to making families and sustaining them, often under difficult personal, economic and social circumstances. We have explored how people as members of families and households manage personal adversity, bring up children, maintain their own and others' health, and provide care to those in poor health or who otherwise need support and care (Knight et al. 2016; Madhavan et al. 2018; Reynolds 2016). We have considered, through the case studies, how local understandings of kinship responsibility and gender usually (but not always) determine who takes on these roles (Schatz & Seeley 2015; Shefer et al. 2008). We have considered how householders seek to balance competing demands; discussed how households may be impacted by changes of their members in health, education and workforce participation; and reflected on how households manage increasing care loads, and the resources on which they draw. From the outset, we have emphasised the impact on families and households of the high levels of circular migration during apartheid and post-apartheid, and the trend to fewer formal marriages and children, and more deaths and outmigration.

Apartheid had profound effects on family organisation and wellbeing, and in the past 25 years, continued economic precarity, political difficulties, HIV and AIDS, and interpersonal conflict likely associated with these pressures have had negative effects on South African households and families. The literature focuses on HIV's impact on families and households, in particular for children (Dawson 2013; Majumdar & Mazaleni 2010; Schatz & Madhavan 2011). There is also a strong literature on gender-based violence and its impact on women and children, again in association with HIV and other social forces (Dunkle et al. 2004; Dworkin et al. 2012). We have chosen, however, not to focus on these aspects; instead, we have widened our scope to cover a range of issues related to family creation, care and health, as kinsfolk balance care demands in the context of household and family change.

Four themes emerge from these chapters: some implicit, others examined explicitly, all worthy of further enquiry. First, although we have not addressed this in a separate chapter, we have reiterated different family forms, differences in gendered partnerships, and the gendering of parental roles. We have not attended to sexuality, however, despite the fact that sexual identity and gender identity inform family-making and household structure, and are manifest in sexual relations, intimacy and vulnerabilities. Gender, age and social context all influence sexual agency, too, and this is part of the context in which families respond to early pregnancy especially, as Nolwazi Mkhwanazi discusses in case study 2.1. Susann Huschke's case study 3.4 is an exception, but sex work is not sexuality; rather, sex work is the one means that enable poor and marginalised women to nurture their children and keep their family intact. We have included some discussions on maternity and paternity, including how paternity is managed in different settings when parents, younger or older, are not together (see case studies 4.1, 4.2 and 4.4), but there is clearly much more that could be explored in this respect.

Second, we have given relatively little space to children, and in so doing we reflect the available literature. The case studies we have included reflect on the role of children in helping to constitute and sustain households and families. Children are the recipients of care, to be sure, but they are also care providers, in everyday life – older children watch out for young siblings, for instance, aiding and comforting them. Children support their parents and grandparents, too, contributing in small ways to the work of maintaining a household, and supporting those with chronic physical or mental-health conditions. In skip-generation households, the grandmother (usually), depending on her age, may have neither time nor energy for certain tasks, such as tending animals, fetching water or fuel, or minding young children. These tasks fall to children of primary- and secondary-school age. Children accompany family members to health centres, help with prescriptions and medication, and may help adults in personal care. They therefore provide emotional, psychological, material and practical care, and in some cases, they take on the full responsibility of maintaining their family in the absence of parents and grandparents.

At the same time, children themselves fall ill, and may experience protracted periods of poor health and/or convalescence. They may be sexually active and may be victims of sexual and other violence; they may experiment with recreational drugs or be involved with gangs; they may be exposed to other risks with profound implications for their maturing and future lives. Yet children and young adults are rarely participants in research, at least in part because of restrictions around the age of consent. Yet if we use this as a reason not to work with children, we ignore critical issues that affect us all; to correct this, we need to engage with children and youth, and build studies with them.

Third, we dealt with femininity implicitly, in association with reproduction and gendered roles, but this boxes this concept in a particular way. We need to further examine how femininity and masculinity, like sexuality and family, are nuanced and fluid, historically and in the present in rural and urban South Africa. There is, in this book, one chapter and various case studies on masculinity, primarily of African men (one, case study 4.4, is on Afrikaner men). In the chapter on men and masculinity, the case-study authors consider paternity in the context of different kinship systems, as well as, one might assume, the desire of some men to be involved in and form a meaningful relationship with their child(ren) if not their children's mother. Throughout the case studies, there is reference to the normative view of men as providers, and the continued gendered division of labour, with the affective and physical labour of care largely being women's work. But men do provide care, for family members and for others. Musariri and Moyer's case study 6.4 highlights how men take on caregiving when family support systems are thin: in one case, when both are migrants and there are no known kin available; in another, when the son-in-law takes on personal care while his wife continues paid employment. The counterpoint to this image is the difficult subject of gender-based violence. As has already been noted, we mentioned this only in passing, except in McBride and Khumalo's case study 4.6, but sexual and other violence against women is pervasive in South Africa. We know less about sexual violence against men, but physical violence among men, including homicide, is not uncommon.

The fourth theme, developed in Chapters 4 and 5, relates to chronic illness, and is concerned with how the chronicity of many infectious and non-communicable conditions is shaped not only by biology and the pathology of the condition, but by the chronicity of social and economic problems. This is central to understanding the complex demands for care that householders and other family members experience. The changing health and wellbeing of one household can profoundly impact on all members of a household. A person may transition from being the carer of others to requiring care themselves, sometimes suddenly, owing to a vehicle or work accident or violence, or due to a sudden change in health (through a stroke, for example). When a person ages, or becomes chronically ill or impaired, often with disease progression, then others may need to make decisions around caregiving, including who might be involved inside or outside a household, and whether they will be paid or unpaid. This, of course, is shaped by household circumstances; paid care is often not affordable. Further, changes in the delivery and receipt of care often occur more organically. Subtle shifts occur over time, with those who have taken on the primary-care roles slowly accruing increasing responsibility. Further, as people transition through different life stages, their roles change, and, as is discussed above, depending on household structure, it may be relatively young children who take on new roles of care. In other cases, care work is reciprocal. Care work may shift between and among individuals over time, even over relatively short periods of time, before the need to give and receive care is constant. In small households, for instance of two people only, where the support of other families is absent, each may seek to care for the other as their health, mobility and capability decline (Nxumalo et al. 2016).

Families provide care both instrumentally and affectively – that is, they care for people they care about – but affective relationships also define what care involves. Occasional support, or checking in, as might be provided by a community health worker or volunteers, is very different from the consistent care work of a co-resident able to provide care on an everyday basis, often all day and all night. This is clear in case study 6.3 by Hellum Braathen and Swartz, who describe the challenges of caring for a household member with a mental-health condition. Under these and similar circumstances, caregiving is constant and may be exhausting. Strained personal and economic resources likely add to this. These strains may contribute to resentment and tensions, at times erupting in violence, but we have little evidence on the neglect and abuse of, and violence against, elders and those with limited capability within households. Moreover, it would be naïve to assume that all householders are willing caregivers, or that all household relationships are caring. That is, people may be in a relationship of pragmatic caregiving and care receipt, but this does not mean that the relationship includes care, affection, or concern.

Connected Lives contributes to our understanding of changes in families. We have brought together scholars working in diverse social-science fields to consider a wide range of health problems and challenges to social wellbeing in urban and rural South Africa. This is a particularly pragmatic way to view the contributions of this book and its case studies. But in drawing together different disciplinary perspectives and authors – from anthropology, sociology, psychology, epidemiology, public health and demography – we have aimed to strengthen conversations around families. These interdisciplinary perspectives complement the differences in focus and accounts, enriching and broadening the accounts of families and households, health and care. And in attending to diversity, we hope, too, that we have celebrated the strengths as well as the challenges of South Africa, and its foundations through the deep social connections that inhere in families and households.

List of contributors

Emily Avera is a PhD candidate in anthropology at Brown University. She holds an MA in anthropology from Leiden University, an MPhil in diversity studies from the University of Cape Town, and a BA in politics from Pomona College. Since 2007, she has conducted social science research focused on transplant and transfusion medicine. Her case study draws on her PhD research, which is focused on blood services in South Africa and is funded by the Fulbright Program and the National Science Foundation. She is a fellow of the Watson Institute's graduate programme in development and is also active in the Science, Technology, and Society programme at Brown.

Deevia Bhana is the DST/NRF South African research chair in gender and childhood sexuality at the University of KwaZulu-Natal. Her research focuses on children's sexual cultures, sexual health and education, significant especially in the context of gender violence, HIV and sexual coercion. She is author of, among other works, *Childhood Sexuality and AIDS Education: The Price of Innocence* (Routledge, 2016) and *Love, Sex and Teenage Sexual Cultures in South Africa* (Routledge, 2018) and is co-editor, with Nolwazi Mkhwanazi, of *Young Families: Gender, Sexuality and Care* (2017).

Deirdre Blackie is a PhD candidate in anthropology at the University of the Witwatersrand. Following a 15-year career in business/brand consulting and change management, she started working with communities concerned with child protection and adoption in 2010. She facilitated the creation of the National Adoption Coalition for South Africa in 2011, and since then her primary focus has been on creating awareness and engaging with communities around child protection challenges. Her case study is based on her master's research that explored the lived experience of child abandonment, following four years of participant observation in communities in and around Johannesburg.

Welmari Bouwer completed her master's in social and psychological research by coursework at the University of the Witwatersrand. She is affiliated to the DST/NRF-Centre of Excellence in Human Development. Her research interests are fatherhood, gender studies, and cross-cultural research.

Stine Hellum Braathen is a research manager at SINTEF in Norway. She has extensive experience conducting research in southern Africa in the fields of disability, mental health and vulnerability, particularly linked to wellbeing, participation and care. She has a PhD from the Department of Psychology, Stellenbosch University. Her thesis focused on aspects of care for people with mental disorders in rural South Africa.

Jenita Chiba works as a researcher at the Centre for Social Development in Africa (CSDA), University of Johannesburg. She is registered for a PhD in social work, with a focus on evaluating a pilot family- and community-based intervention. Her work at the CSDA is largely related to family contexts, family functioning, and exploring supportive programmes for Child Support Grant families, with the aim of enhancing child-wellbeing outcomes. Her case study, co-authored with Tessa Hochfeld and Leila Patel, draws on her current PhD work.

Gabby S. Dlamini is a social anthropology PhD candidate at the University of the Witwatersrand. Her current research focuses on social media, the online creation of material and immaterial value, and personhood. Her master's thesis, 'Living Quietly', was on Swazi middle-class migrants in South Africa, and prior to this, her honours thesis was on *bantfu bentsaba*, who perform royal funeral rites in Swaziland. These research studies frame her broader interests in belonging, relationships, and representation of offline and online human communities in southern Africa.

Casey Golomski holds a PhD and is assistant professor of anthropology and core faculty in women's and gender studies at the University of New Hampshire and a visiting researcher at the University of the Witwatersrand. As a cultural and medical anthropologist, he has conducted field research on death, dying, and ageing, ritual and religion, gender, and healthcare in eSwatini and South Africa. He is the author of articles in *Culture, Health & Sexuality, Medical Anthropology,* and *American Ethnologist,* and the book *Funeral Culture: AIDS, Work, and Cultural Change in an African Kingdom* (2018).

Ntombizonke A. Gumede is a researcher in the Human and Social Development (HSD) research programme of the Human Sciences Research Council (HSRC) in Pretoria, and a PhD candidate at the Critical Studies in Sexualities and Reproduction programme at Rhodes University. Her areas of research specialisation include family, sexual and reproductive health, justice and freedom; participatory action methodologies (quantitative and qualitative), social demography and epidemiology; and belonging, mobility, media, heritage and redress.

Tessa Hochfeld was an associate professor at the Centre for Social Development in Africa, at the University of Johannesburg. She held a PhD in development studies from the University of the Witwatersrand. Tessa's research was built on her background in social development, social protection, social policy and welfare services. Her interest in families related especially to social protection systems and welfare services. She died, tragically, on 17 August 2019.

Rebecca Hodes is the director of the AIDS and Society Research Unit (University of Cape Town), and a research associate of the Department of Social Policy and Intervention (Oxford University). Her work focuses on science, race and sex in the history of South Africa. She is a medical historian, and co-principal investigator of the Mzantsi Wakho study, about the health of 'born free' adolescents in the Eastern Cape. Hodes is interested in the methodological and ethical complexities of integrating quantitative, qualitative and participatory research.

Susann Huschke is an anthropologist and a postdoctoral research fellow at the University of Limerick, researching women's mental health during pregnancy, birth and postpartum. She spent two years as a postdoctoral research fellow in the School of Public Health at the University of the Witwatersrand, conducting a participatory arts-based project on the health and wellbeing of sex workers in Soweto. She has also conducted research in Germany on undocumented migration and migrants' access to healthcare, and in Northern Ireland on sex work, policy and moralities.

Cheyenne Jordaan is a master's candidate in social anthropology at the University of the Witwatersrand. Her academic interests are in pregnancy and childbirth, with past research for her honours degree focusing on private antenatal classes and her current master's research on birth clinics and the experiences of midwives and women in the private healthcare sector. She has also worked with Susann Huschke on the struggles of sex workers in South Africa.

Mzwakhe Khumalo is project coordinator on the Sonke CHANGE Trial, a cluster randomised trial testing a community-mobilisation intervention aiming to prevent violence against women in Diepsloot. He has been with Sonke Gender Justice for seven years, and has led a number of programmes focused on working with men and boys to address gender-based violence and HIV prevention. Previously he was involved in the Men As Partners programme.

Susan Levine holds a PhD and is associate professor of anthropology in the School of African and Gender Studies, Anthropology and Linguistics at the University of Cape Town. She began her career as an anthropologist at the height of AIDS denialism in South Africa, when she joined the national struggle for HIV and AIDS awareness. She is author of *Children of a Bitter Harvest* (2013) and editor of *Medicine and the Politics of Knowledge* (2012), a book that focuses on the ways in which medical diagnoses are produced and interpreted by people in southern Africa, Latin America, China, and India.

Edmond Madhuha is a PhD candidate in health sociology at the University of the Witwatersrand. His current research interests are centred on tuberculosis, masculinities and the health-seeking behaviours of men. His MA thesis, 'The (human) body is like a car – it needs service', explored the relationship between masculinity and health among African working-class men in South Africa. His honours research, undertaken through the University of Johannesburg, was on perceptions of students about absent fatherhood in South Africa.

Ziyanda Majombozi is a lecturer in the Department of Anthropology and Archaeology at the University of Pretoria. She is also a PhD candidate at the University of the Witwatersrand. Her master's research explored women's experiences of infant feeding and, prior to that, her honours looked at how mothers navigate childcare when they are infected with TB. These studies have framed her broader research interests on maternal health, pregnancy, childbirth, childcare, infant feeding and families.

Monde Makiwane is an NRF-rated scientist who is currently in the Human and Social Development (HSD) research programme of the Human Sciences Research Council (HSRC) in Pretoria as a chief research specialist. He also holds a position at North-West University as an extraordinary professor. His areas of research interest include intergenerational relations, ageing, youth, teenage sexuality, fertility, social security and migration.

Mzolisi Makiwane is a BA graduate with a postgraduate degree in education. He has worked as a teacher and a principal in a number of primary and high schools, and is also a mathematics tutor for secondary school learners. He is also a writer, a dramatist and a titled public speaker. In 1980 Mzolisi wrote a popular play, *The Naked Family*, which toured throughout the Eastern Cape in 1983. Mzolisi is a literary activist who is actively promoting reading among primary and high school learners by coordinating literacy festivals.

Lenore Manderson is distinguished professor of public health and medical anthropology in the School of Public Health at the University of the Witwatersrand, with affiliations with Brown and Monash universities. Her research and publications focus on chronic and infectious disease and social circumstance, with attention to how access to technology unequally interacts and impacts on chronic conditions. She also works on questions of climate change, adaptation and advocacy. She edits the journal *Medical Anthropology*, and is founding editor of a monograph series, *Medical Anthropology: Health, Inequality and Social Justice* (Rutgers University Press).

Lebohang Masango is a poet, and has a social anthropology master's degree from the University of the Witwatersrand. Her research interests are youth, romantic relationships and mobile phones. Her current work focuses on how young, digitally connected African women in Johannesburg are subverting 'sugar daddy' relationship modes in order to curate their experiences of love, intimacy and sex. Lebo is also a freelance writer and social commentator with interests in gender, race and popular culture.

Ruari-Santiago McBride is an Irish Research Council fellow and Marie Skłodowska-Curie fellow at the University of Limerick. He leads a project entitled Researching and Advocating for Quality Education: Achieving Equality for Transgender and Gender Diverse Youth in Schools. From 2015 to 2017 he spent two years as a postdoctoral research fellow in the School of Public Health at the University of the Witwatersrand, where he conducted an ethnographic process evaluation of the Sonke CHANGE Trial (a cluster randomised community mobilisation intervention to prevent violence against women in a South African township). His research interests are the intersections of gender, education, health, and justice.

Kathleen Lorne McDougall has been researching perinatal risk management in Cape Town since 2014, as part of the Anthropology of the First 1 000 Days research cluster in the School of African and Gender Studies, Anthropology and Linguistics at the University of Cape Town. Her postdoctoral project has been funded by the National Research Foundation and the Mellon Foundation. She completed her PhD in anthropology from the University of Chicago in 2013, funded by the Wenner-Gren Foundation and the Social Sciences Research Council.

Sonja Merten is a senior public health researcher at the Swiss Tropical and Public Health Institute. Her interests include the household and family as sites where caregiving and care-seeking are negotiated. Over the last fifteen years she has led several research projects on questions around equity in access to health services in various African countries, including on HIV-related care in Zambia, social protection in maternal health in Kenya and in the DRC, and adolescent sexual and reproductive health in the DRC, Rwanda and Burundi.

Nolwazi Mkhwanazi has a PhD in social anthropology from the University of Cambridge (2005), focusing on early childbearing to examine gender and generational relationships in a South African urban township. She is a senior lecturer in anthropology at the University of the Witwatersrand, and presently a senior researcher and director of the Medical Humanities programme at WISER (Wits Institute for Social and Economic Research). Her research interests revolve around youth, gender and reproductive health issues. She is co-editor, with Deevia Bhana, of *Young Families: Gender, Sexuality and Care* (2017).

Langelihle Mlotshwa has conducted research on public health issues in rural and urban South Africa for almost a decade. For her contribution to this book, she draws on her doctoral research, co-supervised by Sonja Merten in the Swiss Tropical and Public Health Institute, Basel, and Lenore Manderson in the School of Public Health, University of the Witwatersrand. Her PhD, conducted in association with the MRC/Wits Developmental Pathways for Health Research Unit, was awarded in 2019. Her interests include pregnancy and the dynamics of the changing family, and how these impact on HIV and AIDS in poor resource settings.

Eileen Moyer holds a PhD and is an associate professor at the University of Amsterdam, specialising in urban and medical anthropology. Her research, which has taken place mainly in eastern and southern Africa, has focused on the entwinement of globalisation, health, and urban identities, with a special interest in the emergence of cosmopolitan socialities related to HIV. In 2015, she was awarded a prestigious European Research Council consolidator grant to research the relationship between global health gender-equality initiatives and transformations in urban African masculinities over the last quarter of a century. Together with Vinh-Kim Nguyen, she also co-edits the open-access journal *Medicine Anthropology Theory*.

Linda Musariri is a PhD candidate at the Amsterdam Institute of Social Science Research, The Netherlands, supervised by Eileen Moyer and by Lenore Manderson in the School of Public Health, University of the Witwatersrand. Her work focuses on how development intervention projects contribute to the shaping of masculinities among migrant men in Johannesburg's CBD. Since 2010, she has worked in the NGO sector focusing mainly on gender equality issues as an activist, and has conducted policy-oriented research on gender-based violence in several countries in the SADC.

Nozipho Mvune is a doctoral candidate at the University of KwaZulu-Natal. She holds a master's degree in gender and education. Her research work focuses on gender and sexuality of young people, with a special interest in rural contexts. Her doctoral research focuses on the experiences of 20 teenage fathers, and how they understand their roles and responsibilities as fathers.

Hanlie Myburgh is a researcher in the social behavioural sciences team at the Desmond Tutu TB Centre at the University of Stellenbosch, and is a PhD candidate in anthropology at the University of Amsterdam. Her research concerns the logics and relationships that govern HIV programme implementation across multiple levels of the health system, from global and national policies to service encounters between health workers and patients, and how the roles and responsibilities of health workers and patients shift as HIV increasingly comes to be understood as a chronic condition.

Mzikazi Nduna hold a PhD and has co-authored 48 peer-reviewed journal articles and 4 book chapters. She has edited a book and three journal special issues. Mzi has research interests in father connections, sexual and reproductive health and rights, gender and gender-based violence, and sexual minorities. She co-edited, with Monde Makiwane and Nene Ernest Khalema, *Children in South African Families: Lives and Times* (2017).

Sara Jewett Nieuwoudt works as a lecturer in the Health and Society Division of the Wits School of Public Health. She coordinates a postgraduate field of study called social and behaviour change communication, which focuses on using a socio-ecological lens to identify and leverage social and individual change processes to address issues of justice and equity. Sara's research interests are in the social determinants of health and gender, specifically as applied to infant feeding and HIV prevention. She is also interested in community-level interventions to shift norms and policy.

Lorena Núñez Carrasco is associate professor in the Department of Sociology at the University of the Witwatersrand. She holds a PhD in medical anthropology from Leiden University. She has conducted extensive research among migrants in both Latin America and southern Africa on topics that intersect culture, health and mobility. She is currently embarked on a comparative project on migration and health between South Africa and Chile, focusing on issues of migration, diversity and race in post-authoritarian societies. She is a co-editor of *Routes and Rites to the City: Mobility, Diversity and Religious Space in Johannesburg* (2017).

Leila Patel is the South African research chair in welfare and social development and the director of the Centre for Social Development in Africa, University of Johannesburg. She played a leading role in the development of welfare policy post-apartheid. Her research interests include social welfare policy, social protection, gender, care, the social services and children and youth. Her recent books are *Development, Social Policy and Community Action: Lessons from below* (with M. Ulriksen, 2017); *Social Welfare and Social Development* (2015); and *Social Protection in Southern Africa* (with J. Midgley and M. Ulriksen, 2014).

Nirvana Pillay is a PhD candidate in the Wits School of Public Health. Her doctoral study is based in Alexandra, Johannesburg, and explores issues of agency and decision-making for young mothers aged 18–20. She is also a consultant in public health and development, with a focus on research, communication and capacity development. Her research interests include maternal and child health, adolescent sexual and reproductive health, the health and wellbeing of farm workers, and migration and health.

Lindsey Reynolds is a research associate in the Department of Sociology and Social Anthropology at Stellenbosch University, and visiting research associate in the Population Studies and Training Center at Brown University. Lindsey is an interdisciplinary researcher, working at the boundaries of anthropology and public health. Her research interrogates tensions inherent in processes of social reproduction and social change in the context of global health research and intervention. She currently consults for the Desmond Tutu TB Centre as social science advisor for HPTN 071 (PopART), a large-scale HIV-prevention trial.

Hanna-Andrea Rother is professor and head of the Environmental Health Division in the School of Public Health and Family Medicine at the University of Cape Town. She holds a PhD in environmental sociology; in this capacity she has made a significant contribution in Africa and globally to the field of environmental health, focusing on children's health, pesticides and other chemicals. This includes her groundbreaking research on the household use of street pesticides in low-income urban communities and resulting child poisonings. Her research, teaching, publications and risk-communication interventions focus on environmental justice, human rights and gender-relevant issues particularly for vulnerable populations in Africa.

Jessica Ruthven undertook her PhD in sociocultural anthropology with a focus in medical anthropology at Washington University in Saint Louis. Her research is at the intersection of HIV and AIDS, gender, the anthropology of performance, creativity, and health communication studies. Her doctoral research, funded by the United States National Science Foundation, was conducted in 2008–2011, and focused on knowledge production and control processes within health-related artistic movements in South Africa. From 2015 to 2017, Jessica was a post-doctoral research fellow in the School of Public Health at the University of the Witwatersrand. She then founded an academic editing and research consulting business and currently works with scholars around the world.

Alison Swartz is a lecturer in the Division of Social and Behavioural Sciences in the School of Public Health and Family Medicine at University of Cape Town (UCT). Her doctoral study, based in Khayelitsha Township in South Africa, investigated the way that young people seek a more adult form of social identity using their gendered identity and sexual partnerships. She has an honours degree in social anthropology, a master's in public health and a PhD in public health from UCT.

Leslie Swartz is a distinguished professor in the Department of Psychology at Stellenbosch University. His work focuses on disability and mental-health issues, focusing largely on southern Africa. He is editor-in-chief of *African Journal of Disability* and associate editor of *Transcultural Psychiatry* and of *International Journal of Disability, Development and Education*.

Elona Toska is a senior research officer at the Centre for Social Science Research and an associate lecturer at the Department of Sociology, University of Cape Town. Her research interests include adolescent sexual and reproductive health, unintended pregnancies, postpartum contraception, and understanding the social and structural factors that underlie HIV infection and poor sexual and reproductive health in adolescents and young people. She works closely with colleagues at UN agencies; South African national and provincial departments of health, social development and basic education; and an inspiring group of adolescents and young people.

Beth Vale is a researcher in humanities at the Mapungubwe Institute for Strategic Reflection (MISTRA). Her research interests span youth body politics, nocturnal cities, HIV interventions, and quotidian productions of sociality as well as power and privilege in South African society. Before joining MISTRA, Beth was a postdoctoral fellow under the NRF chair in local histories, present realities at the University of the Witwatersrand. She has a DPhil from the University of Oxford, for which she investigated the medication-taking practices of HIV-positive adolescents in the Eastern Cape.

Anna Versfeld's PhD in medical anthropology, from the University of Cape Town, focused on the nexus of tuberculosis and substance use in patients accessing public healthcare facilities. This work built on previous research on female methamphetamine users in Cape Town. She currently consults on research and programme implementation related to infectious disease and key populations. Much of her time is spent working with the non-profit organisation TB/HIV Care, where she largely focuses on training people who use drugs to conduct critical, qualitative research related to drug use.

Lario Viljoen is currently pursuing a PhD in the Department of Sociology and Social Anthropology at Stellenbosch University. She also works as a researcher on a major HIV-prevention trial at the Desmond Tutu TB Centre at Stellenbosch. Her PhD focuses on gender, relationship dynamics, intimacy and health narratives in the context of HIV-prevention trials.

References

Adeniyi OV, Ajayi AI, Selanto-Chairman N, Ter Goon D, Boon G, Fuentes YO, Hofmeyr GJ, Avramovic G, Garty C & Lambert J, on behalf of the East London Prospective Cohort Study (ELPCS) Group (2017) Demographic, clinical and behavioural determinants of HIV serostatus nondisclosure to sex partners among HIV-infected pregnant women in the Eastern Cape, South Africa. *PLOS One* 12(8): e0181730

Ahlin T (2018) Only near is dear? Doing elderly care with everyday ICTs in Indian transnational families. *Medical Anthropology Quarterly* 32(1): 85–102

Akyüz A, Yavan T, Şahiner G & Kiliç A (2012) Domestic violence and woman's reproductive health: A review of the literature. *Aggression and Violent Behavior* 17(6): 514–518

Andaya E (2019) Race-ing time: Clinical temporalities and inequality in public prenatal care. *Medical Anthropology* 38(8): 651–663

Ardington C, Branson N, Lam D, Leibbrandt M, Marteleto L, Menendez A, Mutevedzi T & Ranchhod V (2012) *Revisiting the 'crisis' in teen births: What is the impact of teen births on young mothers and their children?* Cape Town: SALDRU, University of Cape Town

AU (African Union) (2003) African Union/HelpAge International (AU/HAI) *Policy Framework and Plan of Action on Ageing*. Nairobi: HAI Africa Regional Development Centre

Avera E (2009) Rationalisation and racialisation in the rainbow nation: Inequalities and identity in the South African Bone Marrow Transplant Network. *Anthropology & Medicine* 16(2): 179–193

Bates B (1992) *Bargaining for life: A social history of tuberculosis, 1876-1938*. Philadelphia: University of Pennsylvania Press

Berry L & Malek E (2017) Caring for children: Relationships matter. In L Jamieson, L Berry & L Lake (Eds) *South African child gauge 2017*. Cape Town: The Children's Institute, University of Cape Town

Bhana D (2005) Violence and the gendered negotiation of masculinity among young black school boys in South Africa. In L Ouzgane & R Morrell (Eds) *African masculinities: Men in Africa from the late nineteenth century to the present*. New York: Palgrave Macmillan

Bhana D (2015) Sex, gender and money in African teenage conceptions of love in HIV contexts. *Journal of Youth Studies* 18(1): 1–15

Bhana D & Anderson B (2013) Desire and constraint in the construction of South African teenage women's sexualities. *Sexualities* 16(5–6): 548–564

Bhana D & Mcambi SJ (2013) When school girls become mothers: Reflections from a selected group of teenage girls in Durban. *Perspectives in Education* 31: 11–19

Bhana D, Morrell R, Shefer T & Ngabaza S (2010) South African teachers' responses to teenage pregnancy and teenage mothers in schools. *Culture, Health & Sexuality* 12(8): 871–883

Bhana D & Nkani N (2014) When African teenagers become fathers: Culture, materiality and masculinity. *Culture, Health & Sexuality* 16(4): 337–350

Bhana D & Pattman R (2011) Girls want money, boys want virgins: The materiality of love amongst South African township youth in the context of HIV and AIDS. *Culture, Health & Sexuality* 13(8): 961–972

Bikaako-Kajura W, Luyirika E, Purcell DW, Downing J, Kaharuza F, Mermin J, Malamba
S & Bunnell R (2006) Disclosure of HIV status and adherence to daily drug regimens
among HIV-infected children in Uganda. *AIDS and Behavior* 10 (Suppl. 7): S85–S93

Blackie D (2014) Sad, bad and mad: Exploring child abandonment in South Africa.
MA dissertation: University of the Witwatersrand

Blackie D (2017) Disrupted families: The social production of child abandonment in urban
Johannesburg. In N Mkhwanazi & D Bhana (Eds) *Young families: Gender, sexuality and care.*
Cape Town: HSRC Press

Blake R (2017) Moral mothers and disobedient daughters: A politics of care and moral
personhood across the generations. In N Mkhwanazi & D Bhana (Eds) *Young families:
Gender, sexuality and care.* Cape Town: HSRC Press

Block E (2014) Flexible kinship: Caring for AIDS orphans in rural Lesotho. *Journal of the Royal
Anthropological Institute* 20(4): 711–727

Block E (2016) Reconsidering the orphan problem: The emergence of male caregivers in Lesotho.
Aids Care 28(Suppl. 4): 30–40

Block E & McGrath W (2019) *Infected kin: Orphan care and AIDS in Lesotho.* New Brunswick:
Rutgers University Press

Bocquier P, Collinson MA, Clark SJ, Gerritsen AAM, Kahn K & Tollman SM (2014) Ubiquitous
burden: The contribution of migration to AIDS and tuberculosis mortality in rural South
Africa. *African Population Studies* 28(1): 691–701

Botha N (2016) Making a baby: A social investigation of assisted reproductive technologies in
and around Pretoria. MSocSci dissertation, Department of Anthropology, University of
Pretoria

Botha N (2017) Mina's story: 'Sick' with child in an Afrikaans-speaking community.
In N Mkhwanazi & D Bhana (Eds) *Young families: Gender, sexuality and care.*
Cape Town: HSRC Press

Button K, Moore E & Seekings J (2018) South Africa's hybrid care regime: The changing and
contested roles of individuals, families and the state after apartheid. *Current Sociology*
66(4): 602–616

Callaway LK, Lust K & McIntyre HD (2005) Pregnancy outcomes in women of very advanced
maternal age. *Australian & New Zealand Journal of Obstetrics & Gynaecology* 45(1): 12–16

Camlin CS, Snow RC & Hosegood V (2013) Gendered patterns of migration in rural South
Africa. *Population, Space and Place* 20(6): 528–551

Chadwick RJ (2016) Obstetric violence in South Africa. *South African Medical Journal*
106(5): 423–424

Chadwick R (2017) Ambiguous subjects: Obstetric violence, assemblage and South African birth
narratives. *Feminism & Psychology* 27(4): 489–509

Chadwick RJ & Foster D (2013) Technologies of gender and childbirth choices: Home birth,
elective caesarean and white femininities in South Africa. *Feminism & Psychology*
23: 317–338

Chikane F (1986) Children in turmoil: The effects of the unrest on township children.
In S Burman & P Reynolds (Eds) *Growing up in a divided society: The contexts of childhood
in South Africa.* Johannesburg: Ravan Press

Chili S & Maharaj P (2015) 'Becoming a father': Perspectives and experiences of young men in
Durban, South Africa. *South African Review of Sociology* 46(3): 28–44

Chopra M, Lawn JE, Sanders D, Barron P, Abdool Karim SS, Bradshaw D, Jewkes R, Abdool Karim Q, Flisher A, Mayosi B, Tollman S, Churchyard G & Coovadia H (2009) Achieving the health Millennium Development Goals for South Africa: Challenges and priorities. *The Lancet* 374(9694): 1023–1031

City of Johannesburg (2005). *Key results: Johannesburg.* Accessed November 2019, http://www.joburg.org.za/corporate_planning/key_results.pdf

City of Johannesburg (2012) *2012/16 integrated development plan: 2013/14 review.* Accessed November 2019, https://www.joburg.org.za/documents_/Documents/Intergrated%20Development%20Plan/2013-16%20IDP%2017may2013%20final.pdf

Clark S, Cotton C & Marteleto LJ (2015) Family ties and young fathers' engagement in Cape Town, South Africa. *Journal of Marriage and Family* 77 (2): 575–589

Clark SJ, Gómez-Olivé FX, Houle B, Thorogood M, Klipstein-Grobusch K, Angotti N, Kabudula C, Williams J, Menken J & Tollman S (2015) Cardiometabolic disease risk and HIV status in rural South Africa: Establishing a baseline. *BMC Public Health* 15(135), doi: 10.1186/s12889-015-1467-1

Clark S, Madhavan S & Kabiru C (2018) Kin support and child health: Investigating two approaches in an African slum. *Social Science Research* 76: 105–119

Clowes L, Ratele K & Shefer T (2013) Who needs a father? South African men reflect on being fathered. *Journal of Gender Studies* 22(3): 255–267

Cluver L, Hodes R, Toska E, Kidia KK, Orkin FM, Sherr L & Meinck F (2015) 'HIV is like a tsotsi. ARVs are your guns': Associations between HIV-disclosure and adherence to antiretroviral treatment among adolescents in South Africa. *AIDS* 29: S57–65

Cluver L, Toska E, Orkin FM, Meinck F, Hodes R, Yakubovich AR & Sherr L (2016) Achieving equity in HIV treatment outcomes: Can social protection improve adolescent ART-adherence in South Africa? *AIDS Care* 28(Suppl. 2): 73–82

Coetzee M (2014) *School quality and the performance of disadvantaged learners in South Africa.* Department of Economics Working Paper No. 22, Stellenbosch University

Cohen WR & Friedman EA (2018) The assessment of labor: A brief history. *Journal of Perinatal Medicine* 46(1): 1–8

Colen S (1986) 'With respect and feelings': Voices of West Indian child care workers in New York City. In JB Cole (Ed.) *All American women: Lines that divide, ties that bind.* New York: Free Press

Collinson MA, Tollman SM & Kahn K (2007) Migration, settlement change and health in post-apartheid South Africa: Triangulating health and demographic surveillance with national census data. *Scandinavian Journal of Public Health* 35(69): Suppl. 77–84, doi: 10.1080/14034950701356401

Collinson MA, White MJ, Bocquier P, McGarvey ST, Afolabi SA, Clark SJ, Kahn K & Tollman SM (2014) Migration and the epidemiological transition: Insights from the Agincourt sub-district of northeast South Africa. *Global Health Action* 7:1, doi: 10.3402/gha.v7.23514

Collinson MA, White MJ, Ginsburg C, Gómez-Olivé FX, Kahn K & Tollman S (2016) Youth migration, livelihood prospects and demographic dividend: A comparison of the Census 2011 and Agincourt Health and Demographic Surveillance System in the rural northeast of South Africa. *African Population Studies* 30(Suppl.2): 2629–2639

Comaroff J (1985) *Body of power, spirit of resistance: The culture and history of a South African people.* Chicago: University of Chicago Press

Conant J (2005) *Pesticides are poison: A community guide to environmental health.* Berkeley: Hesperian Foundation

Connell RW (2005) *Masculinities* (2nd ed.) Berkeley: University of California Press

Connell RW & Messerschmidt JW (2005) Hegemonic masculinity: Rethinking the concept. *Gender & Society* 19(6): 829–859

Coovadia H, Jewkes R, Barron P, Sander D & McIntyre D (2009) The health and health system of South Africa: Historical roots of current health challenges. *The Lancet* 374(9692): 817–834

Cornell D & Van Marle K (2015) Ubuntu feminism: Tentative reflections. *Verbum et Ecclesia* 36(2): 1–8

D'Agostino G, Scarlato M & Napolitano S (2018) Do cash transfers promote food security? The case of the South African Child Support Grant. *Journal of African Economies* 27(4): 430–456

Dahl B (2016) The drama of de-orphaning: Botswana's old orphans and the rewriting of kinship relations. *Social Dynamics* 42(2): 289–303

Dartnall E & Jewkes R (2013) Sexual violence against women: The scope of the problem. *Best Practice and Research Clinical Obstetrics and Gynaecology* 27(1): 3–13

Davies N & Eagle G (2013) Conceptualising the paternal function: Maleness, masculinity, or thirdness? *Contemporary Psychoanalysis* 49(4): 559–585

Davis D (2019) Obstetric racism: The racial politics of pregnancy, labor, and birthing. *Medical Anthropology* 38(7): 560–573

Davis-Floyd R (1992) *Birth as an American Rite of Passage*. Berkeley: University of California Press

Dawson H (2013) HIV/AIDS, the erosion of social capital and the collapse of rural livelihoods in the Nkomazi district of South Africa. *African Journal of AIDS Research* 12(4): 185–194

Deist M & Greeff AP (2017) Living with a parent with dementia: A family resilience study. *Dementia* 16(1): 126–141

Delius P & Glaser C (2002) Sexual socialisation in South Africa: A historical perspective. *African Studies* 61(1): 27–54

Devereux S (2019) Violations of farm workers' labour rights in post-apartheid South Africa. *Development Southern Africa*. doi: 10.1080/0376835X.2019.1609909

Di Stasi A, Milton DR, Poon LM, Hamdi A, Rondon G, Chen J, Pingali SR, Konopleva M, Kongtim P, Aoulsi A, Qazilbash MH, Ahmed S, Bashir Q, Al-atrash G, Oran B, Hosing CM, Kebriaei P, Popat U, Shpall EJ, Lee DA, de Lima M, Rezvani K, Khouri IF, Champlin RE & Ciurea SO (2014) Similar transplantation outcomes for acute myeloid leukemia and myelodysplastic syndrome patients with haploidentical versus 10/10 human leukocyte antigen–matched unrelated and related donors. *Biology of Blood and Marrow Transplantation* 20(12): 1975–1981, doi: 10.1016/j.bbmt.2014.08.013

DoE (Department of Education, South Africa) (2007) *Measures for the prevention and management of learner pregnancy*. Pretoria: Department of Education

DoH (Department of Health, South Africa) (2016) *Implementation of the Universal Test and Treat Strategy for HIV positive patients and differentiated care for stable patients*. Circular. Pretoria: Department of Health

DoH (2017). *Health services*. Accessed August 2019, http://www.health.gov.za/

DoH, UNFPA, Hodes R & Cluver L (2017) *National adolescent and youth national policy 2017*. Pretoria: Department of Health

Doherty T, Chopra M, Nkonki L, Jackson D & Persson L (2006) A longitudinal qualitative study of infant-feeding decision making and practices among HIV-positive women in South Africa. *Journal of Nutrition* 136(9): 2421–2426

DoSD (Department of Social Development, South Africa) (2002) *Plan of action on aging.* Pretoria: South Africa Department of Social Development

Du Plessis L, Peer N, Honikman S & English R (2016) Breastfeeding in South Africa: Are we making progress? In A Padarath, JF King, E Mackie & J Casciola (Eds) *South African Health Review.* Durban: Health Systems Trust

Dulitzki M, Soriano D, Schiff E, Chetrit A, Mashiach S & Seidman DS (1998) Effect of very advanced maternal age on pregnancy outcome and rate of cesarean delivery. *Obstetrics and Gynecology* 92(6): 935–939.

Dunkle KL, Jewkes RK, Brown HC, Gray GE, McIntryre JA & Harlow SD (2004) Gender-based violence, relationship power, and risk of HIV infection in women attending antenatal clinics in South Africa. *The Lancet* 363(9419): 1415–1421

Dunkle KL, Jewkes RK, Nduna M, Levin J, Jama N, Khuzwayo N, Koss MP & Duvvury N (2006) Perpetration of partner violence and HIV risk behaviour among young men in the rural Eastern Cape, South Africa. *AIDS* 20(16): 2107–2114

Dworkin SL, Colvin CJ, Hatcher A & Peacock D (2012) Men's perceptions of women's rights and changing gender relations in South Africa: Lessons for working with men and boys in HIV and antiviolence programs. *Gender and Society* 26(1): 97–120

Enderstein AM & Boonzaier F (2013) Narratives of young South African fathers: Redefining masculinity through fatherhood. *Journal of Gender Studies* 24(5): 512–527

Farmer P (1996) On suffering and structural violence: A view from below. *Daedalus* 125(1): 261–283

Freedman LP (2016) Implementation and aspiration gaps: Whose view counts? *The Lancet* 388(10056): 2968–2069

Freeman MC (2018) Global lessons for deinstitutionalisation from the ill-fated transfer of mental health-care users in Gauteng, South Africa. *Lancet Psychiatry* 5(9): 765–768.

Gari S, Malungo RSJ, Martin-Hilber A, Musheke M, Schindler C & Merten S (2013) HIV testing and tolerance to gender based violence: A cross-sectional study in Zambia. *PLOS ONE* 8(8): e71922

Gaziano TA, Abrahams-Gessel S, Gómez-Olivé FX, Wade A, Crowther NJ, Alam S, Manne-Goehler J, Kabadula CW, Wagner R, Rohr J, Montana L, Kahn K, Bärnighausen TW, Berkman LF & Tollman S (2017) Cardiometabolic risk in a population of older adults with multiple co-morbidities in rural South Africa: The HAALSI (Health and Aging in Africa: Longitudinal studies of INDEPTH communities) study. *BMC Public Health* 17(1): 206, doi: 10.1186/s12889-017-4117-y

George S & McGrath N (2019) Social support, disclosure and stigma and the association with non-adherence in the six months after antiretroviral therapy initiation among a cohort of HIV-positive adults in rural KwaZulu-Natal, South Africa. *Aids Care* 31(7): 875–884

Gibbs A, Jewkes R & Sikweyiya Y (2018) 'I tried to resist and avoid bad friends': The role of social contexts in shaping the transformation of masculinities in a gender transformative and livelihood strengthening intervention in South Africa. *Men and Masculinities* 21(4): 501–520

Gill L (2007) Postfeminist media culture: Elements of a sensibility. *European Journal of Cultural Studies* 10(2): 147–166

Ginsburg F & Rapp R (Eds) (1995) *Conceiving the new world order: The global politics of reproduction.* Berkeley: University of California Press

Goldstein DM & Hall K (2015) Mass hysteria in Le Roy, New York: How brain experts materialised truth and outscienced environmental inquiry. *American Ethnologist* 42(4): 640–657

Golomski C (2016) Outliving love: Marital estrangement in an African insurance market. *Social Dynamics* 42(2): 304–320

Gómez-Olivé FX, Thorogood M, Bocquier P, Mee P, Kahn K, Berkman L & Tollman S (2014) Social conditions and disability related to the mortality of older people in rural South Africa. *International Journal of Epidemiology* 43(5): 1531–1541

Goodley D & Swartz L (2016) The place of disability. In S Grech & K Soldatic (Eds) *Disability in the Global South: The critical handbook*. New York: Springer

Gorman-Smith D, Feig L, Cosey-Gay F & Coeling M (2014) Strengthening families and communities to prevent youth violence: A public health approach. *Children's Legal Rights* 34(3): 265–277

Gouws E & Williams BG (2016) Age-mixing and the incidence of HIV among young women. *The Lancet HIV* 4(1): PE6–E8

Granich R, Gilks C, Dye C, De Cock K & Williams B (2009) Universal voluntary HIV testing with immediate antiretroviral therapy as a strategy for elimination of HIV transmission: A mathematical model. *The Lancet* 373(9657): 48–57

Grove N & Zwi AB (2006) Our health and theirs: Forced migration, othering, and public health. *Social Science & Medicine* 62(8): 1931–1942

Hall K, Linda R, Mokomane K & Lake L (Eds) (2018) *South African child gauge 2018*. Cape Town: The Children's Institute, University of Cape Town

Hall K & Mokomane Z (2018) The shape of families and households: A demographic overview. In K Hall, L Richter, Z Mokomane & L Lake (Eds) *South African child gauge 2018*. Cape Town: Children's Institute, University of Cape Town

Hayes R, Ayles H, Beyers N, Sabapathy K, Floyd S, Shanaube K, Bock P, Griffith S, Moore A, Watson-Jones D, Fraser C, Vermund SH & Fidler S (2014) HPTN 071 (PopART): Rationale and design of a cluster-randomised trial of the population impact of an HIV combination prevention intervention including universal testing and treatment – a study protocol for a cluster randomised trial. *Trials* 15: 57, doi: 10.1186/1745-6215-15-57

Hausmann-Muela S, Muela Ribera J & Nyamongo I (2003) *Health-seeking behaviour and the health system response*. Disease Control Priorities Project Working Paper No. 14

He W, Goodkind D & Kowal P (2016) *An aging world: 2015*, Washington: US Census Bureau and National Institute on Aging, National Institutes of Health

Heinrich C, Hoddinott J, Samson M, MacQuene K, Van Niekerk I & Renaud B (2012) *The South African Child Support Grant impact assessment*. Pretoria: UNICEF, Department of Social Development, and South African Social Security Agency

Hodes R, Doubt J, Toska E, Vale B, Zungu M & Cluver L (2018) The stuff that dreams are made of: HIV-positive adolescents' aspirations for development. *Journal of the International AIDS Society* 21(S1): e25057

HSRC (Human Sciences Research Council) (2012) Study on global ageing and adult health (SAGE), *Wave 1: South Africa National Report*. Geneva: World Health Organization

Hunter M (2005) Cultural politics and masculinities: Multiple partners in historical perspective in KwaZulu-Natal. *Culture, Health & Sexuality* 7(3): 209–223

Hunter M (2010) *Love in the time of AIDS: Inequality, gender, and rights in South Africa*. Bloomington: Indiana University Press

Huschke S (2016) Victims without a choice? A critical view on the debate about sex work in Northern Ireland. *Sexualities Research and Social Policy* 14(2): 192–205

Huschke S (Ed.) (2017) *Know my story: A participatory arts based project.* Accessed November 2019, https://issuu.com/move.methods.visual.explore/docs/kms_final_e-book__11_may_2017__300d

Huschke S & Dlamini Z (2017) A sex worker's view on South Africa's latest plans to beat HIV. *The Conversation.* Accessed November 2019, https://theconversation.com/a-sex-workers-view-on-South-Africas-latest-plans-to-beat-HIV-79355

Hyslop J (2005) Shopping during a revolution: Entrepreneurs, retailers and 'white' identity in the democratic transition. *Historia* 50(1): 173–190

Jacobsson B, Ladfors L & Milsom I (2004) Advanced maternal age and adverse perinatal outcome. *Obstetrics and Gynecology* 104(4): 727–733

James D (2014) *Money from nothing: Indebtedness and aspiration in South Africa.* Stanford: Stanford University Press

James S, Van Rooyen D & Strumpher J (2012) Experiences of teenage pregnancy among Xhosa families. *Midwifery* 28(2): 190–197

Jeffreys S (1997) *The idea of prostitution.* North Melbourne: Spinifex

Jewett Nieuwoudt S (2019) Starting well: Infant feeding practices in the first six months, Soweto, South Africa. PhD dissertation, University of the Witwatersrand

Jewkes R (2005) Non-consensual sex among South African youth: Prevalence of coerced sex and discourses of control and desire. In SJ Jeejobhoy, I Shah & S Thapa (Eds) *Sex without consent: Young people in developing countries.* London: Zed Books

Jewkes R, Abrahams N & Mvo Z (1998) Why do nurses abuse patients? Reflections from South African obstetric services. *Social Science & Medicine* 47(11): 1781–1795

Jewkes R, Dunkle K, Nduna M & Shai N (2010) Intimate partner violence, relationship power inequity, and incidence of HIV infection in young women in South Africa: A cohort study. *The Lancet* 376(9734): 41–48

Jewkes R, Morrell R, Hearn J, Lundqvist E, Blackbeard D, Lindegger G, Quayle M, Sikweyiya Y & Gottzén L (2015) Hegemonic masculinity: Combining theory and practice in gender interventions. *Culture, Health & Sexuality* 17(Suppl. 20): 96–111

Jewkes R, Vundule C, Maforah F & Jordaan E (2001) Relationship dynamics and teenage pregnancy in South Africa. *Social Science & Medicine* 52(5):733–744

Johnson-Hanks J (2002) On the limits of life stages in ethnography: Toward a theory of vital conjunctures. *American Anthropologist* 104(3): 865–880

Jordan B (1978) *Birth in four cultures.* Montreal, QC: Eden Press Women's Publications.

Kahn K, Collinson MA, Gómez-Olivé FX, Mokoena O, Twine R, Mee P, Afolabi SA, Clark BD, Kabudula CW, Khosa A, Khoza S, Shabangu MG, Silaule B, Tibane JB, Wagner RG, Garenne ML, Clark SJ & Tollman SM (2012) Profile: Agincourt Health and Socio-demographic Surveillance System. *International Journal of Epidemiology* 41(4): 988–1001, doi: 10.1093/ije/dys115

Kamwangamalu NM (1999) Ubuntu in South Africa: A sociolinguistic perspective to a pan-African concept. *Critical Arts* 13(2): 24–41

Kaufman M (1993) *Cracking the armour: Power, pain and the lives of men.* Toronto: Viking

Kidia KK, Mupambireyi Z, Cluver L, Ndhlovu CE, Borok M & Ferrand RA (2014) HIV status disclosure to perinatally-infected adolescents in Zimbabwe: A qualitative study of adolescent and healthcare worker perspectives. *PLOS One* 9(1): e87322

Kittay EF, Jennings B & Wasunna AA (2005) Dependency, difference and the global ethic of longterm care. *Journal of Political Philosophy* 13(4): 443–469

Kline W (2019) *Coming home: How midwives changed birth.* New York: Oxford University Press

Knight L, Hosegood V & Timaeus IM (2016) Obligation to family during times of transition: Care, support and the response to HIV and AIDS in rural South Africa. *AIDS Care* 28(Suppl. 4): 18–29

Koenig-Visagie LH & Van Eeden J (2013) Gendered representations of fatherhood in contemporary South African church imagery from three Afrikaans corporate churches. *Verbum et Ecclesia* 34(1): 1–12

Kohler KC, Coetzee BJ & Lochner C (2018) Living with obsessive-compulsive disorder (OCD): A South African narrative. *International Journal of Mental Health Systems* 12: 73, doi: 10.1186/s13033-018-0253-8

Langa M (2010) Adolescent boys' talk about absent fathers. *Journal of Psychology in Africa* 20(4): 519–526

Laopaiboon M, Lumbiganon P, Intarut N, Mori R, Ganchimeg T, Vodel JP, Souza JP, Gülmezoglu AM, on behalf of the WHO Multicountry Survey on Maternal Newborn Health Research Network (2014) Advanced maternal age and pregnancy outcomes: A multicountry assessment. *BJOG: An International Journal of Obstetrics and Gynaecology* 121(s1): 49–56

Leclerc-Madlala S (2003) Transactional sex and the pursuit of modernity. *Social Dynamics* 29(2): 213–233

Leclerc-Madlala S (2008) Age-disparate and intergenerational sex in southern Africa: The dynamics of hypervulnerability. *AIDS* 22: S17–S25

Leclerc-Madlala S (2009) Cultural scripts for multiple and concurrent partnerships in southern Africa: Why HIV prevention needs anthropology. *Sexual Health* 6(2): 103–110

Levitt NS, Steyn K, Dave J & Bradshaw D (2011) Chronic noncommunicable diseases and HIV–AIDS on a collision course: Relevance for health care delivery, particularly in low-resource settings – insights from South Africa. *American Journal of Clinical Nutrition* 94(6): 1690–1696

London L (2005) Editorial: Childhood pesticide poisoning: A clarion call for action on children's vulnerability. *South African Medical Journal* 95(9): 673–674

Lori JR & Boyle JS (2015) Forced migration: Health and human rights issues among refugee populations. *Nursing Outlook* 63(1): 68–76

Lundgren R & Amin A (2015) Addressing intimate partner violence and sexual violence among adolescents: Emerging evidence of effectiveness. *Journal of Adolescent Health* 56(1): s42–50

Luyt R (2012) Constructing hegemonic masculinities in South Africa: The discourse and rhetoric of heteronormativity. *Gender and Language* 6(1): 47–77

Lynch I & Maree DJF (2013) Negotiating heteronormativity: Exploring South African bisexual women's constructions of marriage and family. *Feminism & Psychology* 23(4): 459–477

Macleod C & Morison T (2015) *Men's pathways to parenthood: Silence and heterosexual gendered norms.* Pretoria: HSRC Press

Macleod CI & Tracey T (2010) A decade later: Follow-up review of South African research on the consequences of and contributory factors in teen-aged pregnancy. *South African Journal of Psychology* 40(1): 18–31

Madhavan S & Brooks A (2016) Family complexity in rural South Africa: Examining dynamism in children's living arrangement and the role of kin. *Journal of Comparative Family Studies* 46(4): 483–498

Madhavan S, Clark S & Hara Y (2018) Gendered emotional support and women's well-being in a low-income urban African setting. *Gender and Society* 32(6): 837–859

Madhavan S & Schatz E (2007) Coping with change: Household structure and composition in rural South Africa, 1992–2003. *Scandinavian Journal of Public Health* 69(Suppl. 1): 85–93

Madhuha E (2017) 'The (human) body is like a car – it needs service': Exploring the factors influencing the health-seeking behaviours of working class men in Modimolle town, Limpopo Province. MA dissertation, University of the Witwatersrand

Magubane B (1979) *The political economy of race and class in South Africa*. New York: Monthly Review Press

Mahon-Daly P & Andrews GJ (2002) Liminality and breastfeeding: Women negotiating space and two bodies. *Health & Place* 8(2): 61–76

Majombozi Z (2015) 'Luring the infant into life': Exploring infant mortality and infant feeding in Khayelitsha Cape Town. MA thesis, University of Cape Town

Majumdar B & Mazaleni N (2010) The experiences of people living with HIV/AIDS and of their direct informal caregivers in a resource-poor setting. *Journal of the International AIDS Society* 13(20), doi: 10.1186/1758-2652-13-20

Makiwane M, Gumede NA, Makoae M & Vawda M (2017) Family in a changing South Africa: Structures, functions and the welfare of members. *South African Review of Sociology* 48(2): 49–69

Makiwane M, Ndinda C & Botsis H (2012) Gender, race and aging in South Africa. *Agenda* 26(4): 15–28

Makiwane M, Schneider M & Gopabe M (2004) *Experiences and needs of older persons in Mpumalanga*. Cape Town: HSRC for the Mpumalanga Department of Health and Social Services

Makombo T (2016) Public health sector in need of an antidote. *Insititute for Race Relations: Fast Facts* 6(298): 6

Manderson L (2011) *Surface tensions: Surgery, bodily boundaries and the social self*. Walnut Creek: Left Coast Press

Manderson L & Block E (Guest Eds.) (2016a) *Social Dynamics 42(2): Kinship and Constellations of Care)*

Manderson L & Block E (2016b) Relatedness and care in southern Africa and beyond. *Social Dynamics* 42(2): 205–217

Manderson L, Block E & Mkhwanazi N (Guest Eds.) (2016) *AIDS Care: Psychological and Socio-medical Aspects of AIDS/HIV 28(Suppl. 4: Responsibility, Intimacy and Care)*

Manderson L & Levine S (2018) Southward focused: Medical anthropology in South Africa. *American Anthropologist* 120(3): 566–569

Manderson L & Warren N (2016) 'Just one thing after another': Recursive cascades and chronic conditions. *Medical Anthropology Quarterly* 30(4): 479–497

Marshall JL, Godfrey M & Renfrew MJ (2007) Being a 'good mother': Managing breastfeeding and merging identities. *Social Science & Medicine* 65(10): 2147–2159

Masango L (2019) Johannesburg love, sex and money: An ethnography of phones and feelings. MA dissertation, University of the Witwatersrand

Masvawure T (2010) 'I just need to be flashy on campus': Female students and transactional sex at a university in Zimbabwe. *Culture, Health & Sexuality* 12(8): 857–870

Mathews H, Burke N & Kampriani E (Eds) (2015) *Anthropologies of cancer in transnational worlds*. London: Routledge

Mattes D (2014) 'Life is not a rehearsal, it's a performance': An ethnographic enquiry into the subjectivities of children and adolescents living with antiretroviral treatment in northeastern Tanzania. *Children and Youth Services* Review 45(S1): 28–37

Mayosi BM & Benatar SR (2014) Health and health care in South Africa – 20 years after Mandela. *New England Journal of Medicine* 371(14): 1344–1353

McCloskey LA (2016) The effects of gender-based violence on women's unwanted pregnancy and abortion. *Yale Journal of Biology and Medicine* 89(2): 153–159

Meinck F, Cluver LD, Boyes ME & Mhlongo EL (2015) Risk and protective factors for physical and sexual abuse of children and adolescents in Africa: A review and implications for practice. *Trauma, Violence, & Abuse* 16(1): 81–107

Membe-Matale S (2015) Ubuntu theology. *The Ecumenical Review* 67(2): 273–276

Mendenhall E & Norris SA (2015) When HIV is ordinary and diabetes new: Remaking suffering in a South African township. *Global Public Health* 10(4): 449–462

Merten S (2008) 'Strategic traditions': Changing livelihoods, access to food and child malnutrition in the Zambian Kafue Flats. PhD dissertation: University of Basel

Metz T (2011) Ubuntu as a moral theory and human rights in South Africa. *African Human Rights Law Journal* 11(2): 532–559

Mfecane S (2008) Living with HIV as a man: Implications for masculinity. *Psychology in Society* 36: 45–59

Mfecane S (2016) '*Ndiyindoda*' [I am a man]: Theorising Xhosa masculinity. *Anthropology Southern Africa* 39(3): 204–214

Miller JP, Perry EH, Price TH, Bolan CD Jr, Karanes C, Boyd TM, Chitphakdithai P & King RJ (2008) Recovery and safety profiles of marrow and PBSC donors: Experience of the National Marrow Donor Program. *Biology of Blood and Marrow Transplantation* 14(9 Suppl.): 29–36

Miller K (2016) *Augustown*. London: Weidenfeld and Nicolson

Mjwara N & Maharaj P (2018) Becoming a mother: Perspectives and experiences of young women in a South African township. *Culture, Health & Sexuality* 20(2): 129–140

Mkhwanazi N (2016) Medical anthropology in Africa: The trouble with a single story. *Medical Anthropology* 35(2): 193–202

Mkhwanazi N (2017) Rethabile's story: To be young, pregnant and black. In N Mkhwanazi and D Bhana (Eds) *Young families: Gender, sexuality and care*. Cape Town: HSRC Press

Mkhwanazi N, Berry L, Makusha T, Blackie D, Manderson L, Hall K & Huijbregts M (2018) Negotiating the care of children and support for caregivers. In K Hall, L Richter, Z Mokomane & L Lake (Eds) *South African child gauge 2018: Collaboration and contestation*. Cape Town: The Children's Institute, University of Cape Town

Mkhwanazi N & Bhana D (Eds) (2017) *Young families: Gender, sexuality and care*. Cape Town: HSRC Press

Mkhwanazi N & Block E (2016) Paternity matters: Premarital childbearing and belonging in Nyanga East and Mokhotlong. *Social Dynamics* 42(2): 273–288

Mlotshwa L, Manderson L & Merten S (2017) Personal support and expressions of care for pregnant women in Soweto, South Africa. *Global Health Action* 10(1): 1–10

Moore E (2013) Transmission and change in South African motherhood: Black mothers in three-generational Cape Town families. *Journal of Southern African Studies* 39(1): 151–170

Morison T, Lynch I & Reddy V (2019) *Queer kinship: South African perspectives on the sexual politics of family-making and belonging*. London: Routledge

Morrell R, Bhana D & Shefer T (2012) *Books and babies: Pregnancy and young parents in schools*. Cape Town: HSRC Press

Morrell R & Jewkes R (2011) Carework and caring: A path to gender equitable practices among men in South Africa? *International Journal for Equity in Health* 10(17), doi: 10.1186/1475-9276-10-1

Morrell R, Jewkes R & Lindegger G (2012) Hegemonic masculinity/masculinities in South Africa: Culture, power, and gender politics. *Men and Masculinities* 15(1): 11–30

Moyo K, Núñez L & Leuta T (2016) (Un)rest in peace: The (local) burial of foreign migrants as a contested process of place making. In M Wilhelm-Solomon, L Núñez, P Kankonde Bukasa & B Malcomess (Eds) *Routes and rites to the city: Mobility, diversity and religious space in Johannesburg*. London: Palgrave Macmillan

Mung EM (2008) Chinese migration and China's foreign policy in Africa. *Journal of Chinese Overseas* 4: 91–109

Mvune N, Bhana D & Mayeza E (2019) *Umhlalaphansi* and *inkwari*: Teenage men's accounts on becoming fathers. *Culture Health & Sexuality* 21(2): 147–159

NACSA (National Adoption Coalition of South Africa) (2017) Child protection week 2017. Unpublished presentation

Naidoo J, Muthukrishna N & Nkabinde R (2019) The journey into motherhood and schooling: Narratives of teenage mothers in the South African context. *International Journal of Inclusive Education*, doi: 10.1080/13603116.2019.1600053

Nduna M & Jewkes R (2012) Denied and disputed paternity in teenage pregnancy: Topical structural analysis of case studies of young women from the Eastern Cape province. *Social Dynamics* 38(2): 314–330

Ngabaza S (2011) Positively pregnant: Teenage women's experiences of negotiating pregnancy with their families. *Agenda* 25(3): 42–51

Ngabaza S & Shefer T (2017) Young mothers parenting at school: Gendered narratives on family and care practices. In N Mkhwanazi & D Bhana (Eds) *Young families: Gender, sexuality and care*. Cape Town: HSRC Press

Nhongo TM (2004) The changing role of older people in African households and the impact of aging on African family structures. Paper presented at 'Aging in Africa' conference, Johannesburg. Accessed November 2019, http://arcHIVe.kubatana.net/docs/HIVaid/helpage_impact_of_ageing_0408.pdf.

Nieuwoudt S & Manderson L (2018) Frontline health workers and exclusive breastfeeding guidelines in an HIV endemic South African community: A qualitative exploration of policy translation. *International Breastfeeding Journal* 13: 20, doi: 10.1186/s13006-018-0164-y

Nkani N (2017) Regulating and mediating fathers' involvement in families: The negotiation of *inhlawulo*. In N Mkhwanazi & D Bhana (Eds) *Young families: Gender, sexuality and care*. Cape Town: HSRC Press

Nxumalo N, Goudge J & Manderson L (2016) Community health workers, recipients' experiences and constraints to care in South Africa – a pathway to trust. *AIDS Care* 28(Suppl. 4): 61–71

Nyblade L, Jain A, Benkirane M, Li L, Lohiniva AL, McLean R, Turan JM, Varas-Diaz N, Citron-Bou F, Guan J, Kwena Z & Thomas W (2013) A brief, standardized tool for measuring HIV-related stigma among health facility staff: Results of field testing in China, Dominica, Egypt, Kenya, Puerto Rico and St. Christopher and Nevis. *Journal of the International AIDS Society* 16(3 Suppl. 2): e18718

Old Mutual (2017) *Savings and investment monitor, July 2017.* Cape Town: Old Mutual Limited. Accessed November 2019, https://http://www.oldmutual.co.za/docs/default-source/personal-solutions/financial-planning/savings-and-monitor/latest-research-results/omsim_2017.pdf

Panday S, Makiwane M, Ranchod C & Letsoala T (2009) *Teenage pregnancy in South Africa: With a specific focus on school-going learners.* Cape Town: HSRC Press

Park Y (2009) *A matter of honour: Being Chinese in South Africa.* Plymouth: Lexington Books

Patel L, Knijn T, Gorman-Smith D, Hochfeld T, Isserow M, Garthe R, Chiba J, Moodley J & Kgaphola I (2017a) *Family Contexts, Child Support Grants and child well-being in South Africa.* Johannesburg: Centre for Social Development in Africa, University of Johannesburg

Patel L, Schmid JE & Venter HJ (2017b) Transforming child and family services in urban communities in South Africa: Lessons from the South. *Child and Family Social Work* 22(1): 451–460

Patel P (2017) Forced sterilisation of women as discrimination. *Public Health Reviews* 38(15), doi: 10.1186/s40985-017-0060-9

Pateman C (1999) What's wrong with prostitution? *Women's Studies Quarterly* 27(12): 53–64

Pauw BA (1963) *The second generation: A study of the family among urbanised Bantu in East London.* Cape Town: Oxford University Press

Pereira RB & Whiteford GE (2013) Understanding social inclusion as an international discourse: Implications for enabling participation. *British Journal of Occupational Therapy* 76(2): 112–115

Persson A (2013) Non/infectious corporealities: Tensions in the biomedical era of 'HIV normalisation'. *Sociology of Health and Illness* 35(7): 1065–1079

Philpott RW (1978) What the community needs – obstetric care. *South African Medical Journal* 54: 831–833

Pickles C (2015) Eliminating abusive 'care': A criminal law response to obstetric violence in South Africa. *SA Crime Quarterly* 54: 5–16

Pillay N (2019) Adjusting aspirations: Exploring agency in early motherhood in urban Johannesburg, South Africa. PhD dissertation, University of the Witwatersrand

Pillay N, Manderson L & Mkhwanazi N (2019) Conflict and care in sexual and reproductive health services for young mothers in urban South Africa. *Culture, Health & Sexuality*, doi: 10.1080/13691058.2019.1606282

Posel D (2010) Races to consume: Revisiting South Africa's history of race, consumption and the struggle for freedom. *Ethnic and Racial Studies* 33(2): 157–175

Posel D & Devey R (2006) The demographics of fathers in South Africa: An analysis of survey data, 1993–2002. In L Richter & R Morrell (Eds) Baba: *Men and fatherhood in South Africa.* Cape Town: HSRC Press

Posel D & Marx C (2013) Circular migration: A view from destination households in two urban informal settlements in South Africa. *Journal of Development Studies* 49(6): 819–831

Posel D, Rudwick R & Casale D (2011) Is marriage a dying institution in South Africa? Exploring changes in marriage in the context of *ilobolo* payments. *Agenda* 25(1): 102–111

Press NA & Browner CH (1994) Collective silences, collective fictions: How prenatal diagnostic testing became part of routine prenatal care. In KH Rothenberg & EJ Thomson (Eds) *Women and prenatal testing: Facing the challenges of genetic technology.* Columbus: Ohio State University Press

Quattrocchi P (2019) Obstetric violence observatory: Contributions of Argentina to the international debate. *Medical Anthropology*, doi: 10.1080/01459740.2019.1609471

Ramlagan S, Matseke G, Rodriguez VJ, Jones DL, Peltzer K, Ruiter RAC & Sifunda S (2018) Determinants of disclosure and non-disclosure of HIV-positive status, by pregnant women in rural South Africa. *SAHARA-J: Journal of Social Aspects of HIV/AIDS* 15(1): 155–163

Raniga T & Mthembu M (2017) Family resilience in low income communities: A case study of an informal settlement in KwaZulu-Natal, South Africa. *International Journal of Social Welfare* 26(3): 276–284

Rapp R (2000) *Testing women, testing the fetus: The social impact of amniocentesis in America.* New York: Routledge

Raymond JM & Zolnikov TR (2018) AIDS-affected orphans in sub-Saharan Africa: A scoping review on outcome differences in rural and urban environments. *AIDS and Behavior* 22(10): 3429–3441

Redfield P (2016) Doctors Without Borders and the global emergency. In L Manderson, E Cartwright & A Hardon (Eds) *The Routledge handbook in medical anthropology.* London: Routledge

Reynolds L (2015) Category and kin in 'crisis': Representations of kinship, care, and vulnerability in demographics and ethnographic research in KwaZulu-Natal, South Africa. *Studies in Comparative International Development* 50: 539–560

Reynolds L (2016) Deciphering the 'duty of support': Caring for young people in KwaZulu-Natal, South Africa. *Social Dynamics* 42(2): 253–272

Richter L, Chikovore J & Makusha T (2010). The status of fatherhood and fathering in South Africa. *Childhood Education* 86(6): 360–365

Richter L & Morrell R (Eds) (2006) *Baba: Men and fatherhood in South Africa.* Cape Town: HSRC Press

Roberts JR & Routt Reigart J (2013) *Recognition and management of pesticide poisonings* (6th edition). Washington: US Environmental Protection Agency. Accessed March 2019, http://www.epa.gov/pesticide-worker-safety/pesticide-poisoning-handbook-complete-document

Roelen K, Delap E, Jones C & Chettri HK (2017) Improving child wellbeing and care in sub-Saharan Africa: The role of social protection. *Children and Youth Services Review* 73: 309–318

Rogan M (2013) Poverty and headship in post-apartheid South Africa, 1997–2006. *Social Indicators Research* 113(1): 491–511

Rogan M (2018) Food poverty, hunger and household production in rural eastern Cape households. *Development Southern Africa* 35(1): 90–104

Rother H (2008) Poverty, pests and pesticides sold on South Africa's streets – Implications for women and health. *Women and Environments International Magazine* 76: 36–43

Rother H (2010) Falling through the regulatory cracks: Street selling of pesticides and poisoning among urban youth in South Africa. *International Journal of Occupational and Environmental Health* 16(2): 202–213

Rother H (2016) Pesticide vendors in the informal sector trading health for income. *NEW SOLUTIONS: A Journal of Environmental and Occupational Health Policy* 26(2): 241–252, doi: 10.1177/1048291116651750

Rothman SM (1995) *Living in the shadow of death: Tuberculosis and the social experience of illness in American History.* Baltimore: Johns Hopkins University Press

Rudwick S & Posel D (2015) Zulu bridewealth (*ilobolo*) and womanhood in South Africa. *Social Dynamics* 41(2): 289–306

Russell M, Cupp PK, Jewkes R, Gevers A, Mathres C, Lefleur-Bellerose C & Small J (2014) Intimate partner violence among adolescents in Cape Town, South Africa. *Prevention Science* 15(3): 283–295

Salo E (2003) Negotiating gender and personhood in the new South Africa. *European Journal of Cultural Studies* 6: 345–365

Sanlam Wealthsmiths (2016) *Benchmark survey 2016. Rethinking retirement through a new dimension*. Research Insights Report. Cape Town: Sanlam

Schatz E (2009) Reframing vulnerability: Mozambican refugees' access to state-funded pensions in rural South Africa. *Journal of Cross-Cultural Gerontology* 24(3): 241–258

Schatz E, Gómez-Olivé FX, Ralston M, Menken J & Tollman S (2012) The impact of pensions on health and wellbeing in rural South Africa: Does gender matter? *Social Science & Medicine* 75(10): 1864–1873

Schatz E & Madhavan M (2011) Headship of older persons in the context of HIV/AIDS in rural South Africa. *African Population Studies* 25(2): 440–456

Schatz E, Madhavan S, Collinson M, Gómez-Olivé FX & Ralston M (2015) Dependent or productive? A new approach to understanding the social positioning of older South Africans through living arrangements. *Research on Aging* 37(6): 581–605

Schatz E, Madhavan S & Williams J (2011) Female-headed households contending with AIDS-related hardship in rural South Africa. *Health & Place* 17(2): 598–605

Schatz E & Ogunmefun C (2007) Caring and contributing: The role of older women in rural South African multi-generational households in the HIV/AIDS era. *World Development* 35(8): 1390–1403

Schatz E & Seeley J (2015) Gender, ageing and carework in East and Southern Africa: A review. *Global Public Health* 10(10): 1185–1200

Schenck R & Blaauw D (2018) Day labourers: A case study of the vulnerability of the social fabric and cohesion in South Africa's informal economy. *Tydskrif Vir Geesteswetenskappe* 58(1): 36–55

Scheper-Hughes N (1992) *Death without weeping: The violence of everyday life in Brazil*. Berkeley: University of California Press

Schneider H, Hlophe H & Van Rensburg D (2008) Community health workers and the response to HIV/AIDS in South Africa: Tensions and prospects. *Health Policy and Planning* 23(3): 179–187

Seidel G (2004) Decisions and advice about infant feeding: Findings from sociological work in KwaZulu-Natal, South Africa. *African Journal of AIDS Research* 3(2): 167–177

Selikow TA & Mbulaheni T (2013) 'I do love him but at the same time I can't eat love': Sugar daddy relationships for conspicuous consumption amongst urban university students in South Africa. *Agenda* 27(2): 86–98

Selin A, DeLong SM, Julien A, MacPhail C, Twine R, Hughes JP, Agyei Y, Hamilton EL, Kahn K & Pettifor A (2019) Prevalence and associations, by age group, of IPV among AGYW in rural South Africa. *SAGE Open* 9(1), doi.org/10.1177/2158244019830016

Sharp LA (2006) *Strange harvest: Organ transplants, denatured bodies and the transformed self*. Berkeley and Los Angeles: University of California Press

Shefer T, Bhana D & Morrell R (2013) Teenage pregnancy and parenting at school in contemporary South African contexts: Deconstructing school narratives and understanding policy implications. *Perspectives in Education* 31: 1–10

Shefer T, Bhana D, Morrell R, Manzini N & Masuka N (2012) 'It isn't easy': Young parents talk of their school experiences. In R Morrell, D Bhana & T Shefer (Eds) *Books and babies: Pregnancy and young parents in schools.* Cape Town: HSRC Press

Shefer T, Crawford M, Strebel A, Simbayi LC, Dwada-Henda N, Cloete A, Kaufman MR & Kalichman SC (2008) Gender, power and resistance to change among two communities in the Western Cape, South Africa. *Feminism and Psychology* 18(2): 157–182

Shenderovich Y, Eisner M, Cluver L, Doubt J, Berezin M, Majokweni S & Murray AL (2018). What affects attendance and engagement in a parenting program in South Africa? *Prevention Science* 19(7): 977–986

Shisana O, Rehle T, Simbayi LC, Zuma K, Jooste S, Zungu N, Labadarios D & Onoya D (2014) *South African national HIV prevalence, incidence and behaviour survey, 2012* Cape Town: HSRC Press

Shope JH (2006) 'Lobola is here to stay': Rural black women and the contradictory meanings of lobola in post-apartheid South Africa. *Agenda* 20(68): 64–72

Singer M (2009) *Introduction to syndemics: A critical systems approach to public and community health.* Chichester: John Wiley and Sons

Singer M, Bulled N, Ostrach B & Mendenhall E (2017) Syndemics and the biosocial conception of health. *The Lancet* 389(10072): 941–945

Singh S & Naicker P (2017) Control as support: Improving the outcomes for teenage mothers. In N Mkhwanazi & D Bhana (Eds) *Young families: Gender, sexuality and care.* Cape Town: HSRC Press

Smit R (2001) The impact of labor migration on African families in South Africa: Yesterday and today. *Journal of Comparative Family Studies* 32(4): 533–548

Squire C (2015) Partial secrets. *Current Anthropology* 56(S12): S201–S210

Stats SA (2016) *Mid-year population estimates, 2015.* Statistical Release P0302. Pretoria: Stats SA

Stats SA (2017) *Poverty trends in South Africa: An examination of absolute poverty between 2006 and 2015,* Statistician-General Report No. 03-10-06. Pretoria: Statistics South Africa

Stats SA (2018) *Statistical release P0302: Mid-year population estimates 2018.* Pretoria: Statistics SA

Stats SA (2019) *Statistical release P0302. Mid-year population estimates 2019.* Pretoria: Stats SA

Steinert JI, Cluver LD, Meinck F, Doubt J & Vollmer S (2018) Household economic strengthening through financial and psychosocial programming: Evidence from a field experiment in South Africa. *Journal of Development Economics* 134: 443–466

Stenglin M & Foureur M (2013) Designing out the fear cascade to increase the likelihood of normal birth. *Midwifery* 29(6): 819–825

Swartz A, Levine S, Rother H & Langerman F (2018) Toxic layering through three disciplinary lenses: Childhood poisoning and street pesticide use in Cape Town, South Africa. *Medical Humanities* 44(4): 247–252

Swartz S & Bhana A (2009) *Teenage tata: Voices of young fathers in South Africa.* Cape Town: HSRC Press

Synergos (2014) *Building social connectedness: A brief guide for practitioners working with children and youth.* Social Connectedness Programme, Johannesburg: Synergos South Africa

Szer J, Elmoazzen H, Fechter M, Hwang W, Korhonen M, Miller J, Mengling T, Shaw B & Stein J (2016) Safety of living donation of hematopoietic stem cells. *Transplantation* 100(6): 1329–1331

Tanner M & Vlassoff C (1998) Treatment-seeking behaviour for malaria: A typology based on endemicity and gender. *Social Science & Medicine* 46(4–5): 523–532

Tolhurst R, Amekudzi YP, Nyonator FK, Squire SB & Theobald S (2008) 'He will ask why the child gets sick so often': The gendered dynamics of intra-household bargaining over healthcare for children with fever in the Volta Region of Ghana. *Social Science & Medicine* 66(5): 1106–1117

Toska E, Cluver L, Hodes R & Kidia KK (2015) Sex and secrecy: How HIV-status disclosure affects safe sex among HIV-positive adolescents. *AIDS Care* 27(Suppl. 1): 47–58

Treves-Kagan S, Steward WT, Ntswane L, Haller R, Gilvydis JM, Gulati H, Barnhart S & Lippman SH (2016) Why increasing availability of ART is not enough: A rapid, community-based study on how HIV-related stigma impacts engagement to care in rural South Africa. *BMC Public Health* 16(87), doi: 10.1186/s12889-016-2753-2

Turner BS (1992) *Regulating bodies: Essays in medical sociology.* London: Routledge

UN (United Nations), Department of Economic and Social Affairs, Population Division (2017) *World population ageing 2017 – Highlights* (ST/ESA/SER.A/397). New York: United Nations, Department of Economic and Social Affairs, Population Division

UNAIDS (Joint United Nations Programme on AIDS/HIV) (2016). *AIDSinfo.* Accessed June 2018, http://AIDSinfo.unAIDS.org/

UNIFEM (United Nations Development Fund for Women) (2011) *Violence against women: Facts and figures.* New York: UNIFEM

Vale B, Cluver L & Hodes R (2017) Negotiations of blame and care among HIV-positive mothers and daughters in South Africa's Eastern Cape. *Medical Anthropology Quarterly* 31(4): 519–536

Vale B & Thabeng M (2016) Redeeming lost mothers: Adolescent antiretroviral treatment and the making of home in South Africa. *Medical Anthropology* 35(6): 489–502

Van den Berg W & Makusha T (2018) *State of South Africa's fathers 2018.* Cape Town: Sonke Gender Justice & Human Sciences Research Council

Van Rensburg AJ, Wouters E, Fourie P, Van Rensburg D & Bracke P (2018) Collaborative mental health care in the bureaucratic field of post-apartheid South Africa. *Health Sociology Review* 27(3): 279–293

Versfeld A (2017) Aliyah's story: Generational change in Manenburg. In N Mkhwanazi & D Bhana (Eds) *Young families: Gender, sexuality and care.* Cape Town: HSRC Press

Vilanculos E & Nduna M (2017) 'The child can remember your voice': Parent–child communication about sexuality in the South African context. *African Journal of AIDS Research* 16(1): 81–89

Viljoen S (2011) 'Papa don't preach': Fatherhood in a South African Christian men's magazine. *Communicatio* 37(2): 308–331

Walker R, Vearey J & Nencel L (2017) Negotiating the city: Exploring the intersecting vulnerabilities of non-national migrant mothers who sell sex in Johannesburg, South Africa. *Agenda* 31(1): 91–103

Walker RJ (2017) 'If this isn't for my children, who is it for?' Exploring experiences of structural violence among migrant mothers who sell sex in Johannesburg. *Families, Relationships and Societies* 6(2): 291–306

Weiss B (2000) Vulnerability of children and the developing brain to neurotoxic hazards. *Environmental Health Perspectives* 108(Suppl. 3): 375–381

WHO (World Health Organization) (2010) *The WHO recommended classification of pesticides by hazard and guidelines to classification 2009.* Geneva: World Health Organization

WHO (World Health Organization) (2017) *Global strategy and action plan on ageing and health.* Geneva: World Health Organization

Wikan U (2013) *Resonance: Beyond the words.* Chicago: University of Chicago Press

Wood K, Lambert H & Jewkes R (2007) 'Showing roughness in a beautiful way': Talk about love, coercion, and rape in South African youth sexual culture. *Medical Anthropology Quarterly* 21(3): 277–300

Wood K, Lambert H & Jewkes R (2008) 'Injuries are beyond love': Physical violence in teenage South Africans' sexual relationships. *Medical Anthropology* 27(1): 43–69

World Bank (2014) *South Africa economic update: Fiscal policy and redistribution in an unequal society.* Washington: World Bank

Zembe-Mkabile W, Surender R, Sanders D, Swart R, Ramokolo V, Wright G & Doherty T (2018) 'To be a woman is to make a plan': A qualitative study exploring mothers' experiences of the Child Support Grant in supporting children's diets and nutrition in South Africa. *BMJ Open* 8(4): e019376

Zulliger R, Abrams EJ & Myer L (2013) Diversity of influences on infant feeding strategies in women living with HIV in Cape Town, South Africa: A mixed methods study. *Tropical Medicine & International Health* 18(12): 1547–1554

Zuma J (2017) *State of the nation address.* Accessed October 2019, https://www.gov.za/speeches/president-jacob-zuma-2017-state-nation-address-9-feb-2017-0000

Index